HEALTH INFORMATICS

AN ADAPTIVE COMMUNICATION TECHNOLOGY FOR FUTURE HEALTHCARE

HEALTH CARE IN TRANSITION

Additional books in this series can be found on Nova's website under the Series tab.

Additional E-books in this series can be found on Nova's website under the E-books tab.

PUBLIC HEALTH IN THE 21ST CENTURY

Additional books in this series can be found on Nova's website under the Series tab.

Additional E-books in this series can be found on Nova's website under the E-books tab.

HEALTH CARE IN TRANSITION

HEALTH INFORMATICS

AN ADAPTIVE COMMUNICATION TECHNOLOGY FOR FUTURE HEALTHCARE

NAVEEN CHILAMKURTI
EDITOR

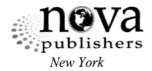

nova
publishers
New York

Copyright © 2013 by Nova Science Publishers, Inc.

For permission to use material from this book please contact us:
Telephone 631-231-7269; Fax 631-231-8175
Web Site: http://www.novapublishers.com

NOTICE TO THE READER

The Publisher has taken reasonable care in the preparation of this book, but makes no expressed or implied warranty of any kind and assumes no responsibility for any errors or omissions. No liability is assumed for incidental or consequential damages in connection with or arising out of information contained in this book. The Publisher shall not be liable for any special, consequential, or exemplary damages resulting, in whole or in part, from the readers' use of, or reliance upon, this material. Any parts of this book based on government reports are so indicated and copyright is claimed for those parts to the extent applicable to compilations of such works.

Independent verification should be sought for any data, advice or recommendations contained in this book. In addition, no responsibility is assumed by the publisher for any injury and/or damage to persons or property arising from any methods, products, instructions, ideas or otherwise contained in this publication.

This publication is designed to provide accurate and authoritative information with regard to the subject matter covered herein. It is sold with the clear understanding that the Publisher is not engaged in rendering legal or any other professional services. If legal or any other expert assistance is required, the services of a competent person should be sought. FROM A DECLARATION OF PARTICIPANTS JOINTLY ADOPTED BY A COMMITTEE OF THE AMERICAN BAR ASSOCIATION AND A COMMITTEE OF PUBLISHERS.

Additional color graphics may be available in the e-book version of this book.

LIBRARY OF CONGRESS CATALOGING-IN-PUBLICATION DATA

ISBN: 978-1-61942-265-0

Published by Nova Science Publishers, Inc. † New York

CONTENTS

PREFACE

The current growth of Internet and communication technologies has given a new dimension to health care system. Using high speed communication networks, physicians are now able to remotely monitor patients and were able to perform some diagnosis also. But, health care industry is very sensitive to communication technologies as quality of service and delay constrains are paramount in this field. As the research in communication has matured in recent years, now the health care industry is moving to another level and is ready to accept Information Technology (IT) as one of its driving tool. Due to recent advances in IT, more and more applications are focusing on providing better communication tools and applications to both physicals and patients. Recent RFID and sensor technologies are also helping health industry in monitoring and diagnosis of patients. Health informatics deals with all information and records related to health care management. More and more countries are implanting health care informatics and are investing in this area for better health of their population. This will not only help them manage public health a better way, but also reduces the cost of manually handling records, patient x-rays so and so forth. Health informatics has wide are of applications and if used properly can benefit world population for better health. In this book we provide more recent wide applications of IT in health industry starting from health care using small sensors such as Body Sensor Networks (BSN), RFID's to more context-aware e-health applications. The book chapters provide a clear picture of recent advances in health informatics with a vision of future applications in this domain. This useful book will enable interested readers, researchers, graduate students to familiarize themselves with the new e-health paradigm and in future to contribute to new advances in this field too.

Chapter 1 - Today, the ubiquity of mobile phones and the growing need for enhanced medical services worldwide provide a unique opportunity to develop various type of mobile healthcare (mHealth) applications and services. In this chapter, the authors introduce the novel concept of cost-effective mobile healthcare, with emphasis on networking and data transfer, to bridge this gap for low-income communities. The targeted system leverages the multiple wireless interfaces on board most mobile phones available today. They aim to develop a ubiquitous healthcare system based on the use of the widespread sensor-rich mobile phones along with emerging wireless-enabled medical devices. The authors begin by presenting the problem of uploading medical data using the "optimal" wireless interface, from a cost perspective. Towards this objective, we present a simple Wireless Interface Selection Algorithm (WISA) which targets the wireless interface yielding minimum cost, depending on the data size, modality and QoS (particularly delay) constraints. Afterwards, they study the problem of cost-effective advisory message dissemination (from the health authorities to a group of co-located mobile phones). This gives rise to an interesting cost-delay trade-off when leveraging the free device-device direct communication interface (e.g., Bluetooth). The authors build a proof-of-concept testbed, coined *CellChek*, which showcases the proposed concepts and algorithms anddemonstrates their operation with exemplary wireless- enabled medical devices, namely pulse oximeter and blood pressure monitor, and plausible use cases. The concepts explored in this chapter along with the proposed schemes and testbed hold great promise for this rapidly growing area of research within the mobile healthcare arena that is of equal importance to developing and developed countries.

Chapter 2 - Mobile devices are becoming more and more popular in a large variety of application domains. In particular, new sensor technologies, powerful mobile devices, and wearable computers in conjunction with wireless communication standards have opened new opportunities in providing customized software solutions. This is particularly relevant in eHealth applications, from pervasive information access in hospital environments to the individual support of patients, both in stationary and home care. Medical professionals are equipped today with much more powerful hardware and software than some years before. By making use of smart sensors and mobile devices for gathering, processing, and analyzing data, medical doctors and nursing staff are able to get access to relevant information (e.g., patient records) anytime and anywhere in a hospital. Similarly, for patients this technology can be used to provide support which is tailored to their particular needs and impairments. All these environments are highly dynamic, due to the inherent mobility of users. Therefore, in order to best serve the individual information needs of the different users in eHealth applications, it is of utmost importance to automatically adapt the underlying IT environment to their context – which might change over time when user context evolves. In a digital home environment, this requires the automatic customization of user interfaces and the context-aware adaptation of monitoring workflows for mobile patients. In a hospital environment, such dynamic adaptations will for instance help physicians to automatically retrieve and present the data they need in their current context, without having them to manually search for relevant information (e.g., on a ward round or in an emergency case). This chapter will give an overview on context-awareness in mobile environments with particular focus on eHealth applications and the special requirements of users in healthcare applications. It will introduce LoCa (a Location and Context-aware eHealth infrastructure), a concrete system that provides a generic software infrastructure, able to dynamically adapt user interfaces and service-based distributed applications (workflows) to the actual context of a user (physician, caregiver, patient, etc.). Furthermore, the chapter will report on the evaluation of the LoCa system based on a prototype system running on smart phones.

Chapter 3 - From the perspective of network design, network patient capacity, which the authors define as the number of patients that one wireless local area network deployment can support, is a critical design criterion and performance metric for wireless healthcare systems. In this chapter, they first introduce the background of wireless healthcare systems, including the motivations, the categories, the architectures, and the challenges of wireless healthcare in-hospital monitoring systems. Building on the specific characteristics of the wireless healthcare monitoring environment, the authors study network patient capacity in view of two particular issues for wireless systems, namely, imperfect channel state information (CSI) and electro-magnetic interference (EMI).

Chapter 4 - Recently there has been an upsurge of research interest on Body Sensor Networks (BSNs). In BSNs, biomedical sensor nodes are deployed in the different parts of the human physiological system. These nodes interconnect to form a network through which vital physiological information sensed by the sensors deployed on the human body are sent to the control center for further processing and patient monitoring. The expeditious advancements in biomedical sensors, low power integrated circuits, short range RF transceivers and low-cost antennas (directional/omni-directional) have helped in the realization of BSNs. Increased network reliability, ease of accessibility, real-time monitoring of patients are fundamental research challenges of concern in BSNs. BSNs have specific characteristics that make them unique over regular Wireless Sensor Networks (WSNs). Unlike regular WSNs, mobility models for BSNs are influenced by the human body movement. The low transmitted power signal of the nodes in BSNs minimizes the risk of health hazards. By having implanted sensors closer to the suspected areas of the human body, it is possible to analyze the information about the chronological state of the different parts of the body through offline or online means, depending upon the severity of the disease affecting the body. For instance, data transaction would be in non-real-time for monitoring the metabolic rate of cells (chemical reaction), insulin/glucagon level in blood, blood pressure, heart-rate, lungs-rate, blood viscosity of an athletic, and can be analyzed using offline techniques. On the contrary, a group of cancerous cells have to be monitored in an online manner. In recent years, many protocols and algorithms have been proposed for BSNs. Some of the popular ones include medium access control (MAC) protocols (e.g., H-MAC and BSN-MAC) and Delay-Tolerant Network (DTN) —in this case Body-DTN— are mostly concerned. In this chapter we review the architecture and protocols for BSNs.

Chapter 5 - Everybody touches the healthcare issues. However, people 65 years and over need more than everyone and three primary forces affect their live: 1) their population increase; 2) they need more healthcare support; and 3) their incomes decrease. Availability of their care in their own homes is imperative because of the economic reasons and their choices where to live. Recent advancement in the information and communication technology are creating a new types of services. For instance, wireless communications and electronics have enabled the development of low-cost sensor networks and they can be employed in smart homes, e-healthcare applications and assisted living services. These statements show that there is a great promise in wireless technology and utilizing it in assisted living might be very beneficial to the elderly people. In this chapter, the authors propose a software architecture called the Location Windows Service (LWS) which integrates the Radio Frequency Identification (RFID) technology and the web service to build an assisted living system for elderly people at home. This architecture monitors the location of elderly people without interfering in their daily activities. Location information messages that are generated as the elderly move from room to room indicate that the elderly person is fit and healthy and going about their normal life. The communication must be timely enough to follow elderly people as they move from room to room without missing a location.

Unacknowledged publishing, subscription filtering and short location change messages are also included in this software model to reduce the network traffic in large homes.

Chapter 6 - This paper examines a wide variety of issues concerning the doctor-patient relation, the medical model, the role of technology in self-care, and the issues of patient empowerment in current healthcare systems. The aim of the paper is to open up a debate concerning many of the background assumptions embedded in the rapidly expanding fields of self-care and home-health care, and to re-shape the role of technology in the design of a truly patient-centred healthcare system.

In: Health Informatics   ISBN: 978-1-61942-265-0
Editor: Naveen Chilamkurti   © 2013 Nova Science Publishers, Inc.

Chapter 1

COST-EFFECTIVE NETWORKING FOR MOBILE HEALTHCARE

Yossuf Khazbak[1], Mostafa Izz[1], Tamer ElBatt[1]
and Moustafa Youssef[2]
[1] Nile University, Egypt
[2] Egypt-Japan University of Science and Technology, Egypt

Today, the ubiquity of mobile phones and the growing need for enhanced medical services worldwide provide a unique opportunity to develop various type of mobile healthcare (mHealth) applications and services. In this chapter, we introduce the novel concept of cost-effective mobile healthcare, with emphasis on networking and data transfer, to bridge this gap for low-income communities. The targeted system leverages the multiple wireless interfaces on board most mobile phones available today. We aim to develop a ubiquitous healthcare system based on the use of the widespread sensor-rich mobile phones along with emerging wireless-enabled medical devices. We begin by presenting the problem of uploading medical data using the "optimal" wireless interface, from a cost perspective. Towards this objective, we present a simple Wireless Interface Selection Algorithm (WISA) which targets the wireless interface yielding minimum cost, depending on the data size, modality and QoS (particularly delay) constraints. Afterwards, we study the problem of cost-effective advisory message dissemination (from the health authorities to a group of co-located mobile phones). This gives rise to an interesting cost-delay trade-off when leveraging the free device-device direct communication interface (e.g., Bluetooth). We build a proof-of-concept testbed, coined *CellChek*, which showcases the proposed concepts and algorithms and demonstrates their operation with exemplary wireless- enabled medical devices, namely pulse oximeter and blood pressure monitor, and plausible use cases. The concepts explored in this chapter along with the proposed schemes and testbed hold great promise for this rapidly growing area of research within the mobile healthcare arena that is of equal importance to developing and developed countries.

1. Introduction

1.1. Motivation

The wireless technology wide proliferation has inspired many novel applications and services that range from social, business, national security, and defense to healthcare-related services [1]. Despite the remarkable progress achieved in several arenas, fully leveraging ubiquitous mobile communications for healthcare services in under-served communities remains a daunting challenge. The recently witnessed convergence of sensing, communications and computing creates ample opportunity for providing secure, reliable and timely tele-health services in general, and mobile healthcare services in particular, for under-served communities around the world where healthcare services are either too costly or not immediately available. This is primarily attributed to the acute shortage of qualified healthcare professionals, and consequently health education and training, and the limited availability of advanced medical equipment in developing countries, among other factors.

On the other hand, the continuously increasing number of mobile subscribers around the world creates ample opportunity for ubiquitous (i.e. anywhere, anytime) healthcare, among other, services. Mobile phones have achieved significant penetration globally, and in developing nations in particular, over the past decade. According to the estimates of the International Telecommunication Union (ITU), there were 5.3 billion mobile subscribers worldwide at the end of 2010, including 3.8 billion in developing countries [2]. Furthermore, access to a mobile network is now available to 90% of the world's population, including 80% of the population living in rural areas. Finally, the numbers of internet-capable mobile phones and devices is rapidly increasing worldwide. For instance, there were 940 million subscriptions to 3G data services worldwide at the end of 2010.

The use of mobile devices to improve healthcare, dubbed "mHealth", has been one of the most prominent areas within the broader emerging field of "mDevelopment" encompassing novel use cases, e.g., mLearning and mCommerce. For instance, mobile devices are transforming lives and accelerating development through a wide range of applications including dissemination of crops and agricultural products' prices, mobile banking, gathering data on disease epidemics, among many others. mHealth includes a breadth of initiatives ranging from treatment adherence to data collection, drug control, supply chain management, and health financing and education. mHealth Education is a rapidly growing area that falls at the intersection of mHealth and mLearning and holds great promise for solving the aforementioned healthcare challenges in developing countries and under-served communities.

The pressing need for healthcare services for low-income communities coupled with the prevailing opportunity presented by the wide proliferation of mobile Internet access set the perfect stage for a new research paradigm which constitutes the subject matter of this chapter, namely cost-effective mobile healthcare. Despite the fact that leveraging mobile phones for mobile healthcare services is not a new concept as evidenced by recent literature [3–12], the emphasis on cost savings as a major design driver, rather than after-the-fact design issue, has not received sufficient attention from the community and remains largely unexplored.

1.2. Contributions

The prime objective of this chapter is to introduce this ripe area of research and shed light on a specific problem within this space, namely cost-effective networking for mHealth. This is achieved via leveraging the multiple radio interfaces available on smart phones today, and soon will be available on a wide range of mobile phones, including low-end phones, thanks to the Very Large Scale Integration (VLSI) industry trends projected by Moore's law. The envisioned cost-effective mobile healthcare system, coined *CellChek*, is not only tailored to overcome a unique set of challenges inherent to mobile phone usage in low-income communities (e.g., expensive data plans, predominantly pre-paid plans, limited public WiFi access) but also poised to effectively exploit a unique set of features inherent to Cellular 3G systems (e.g., free incoming calls, inexpensive SMS service). *CellChek* is envisioned to leverage a plethora of sensing modalities ranging from wireless-enabled on-body medical devices (e.g., blood pressure, pulse oximeter and ECG) to mobile phone sensors (e.g., accelerometer, GPS and camera).

Our major contribution in the cost-effective mobile healthcare arena, presented in this chapter, is three-fold. First, we introduce the novel concept of cost-effective data transfer for remote patient monitoring and medical advisory dissemination tailored to address the challenges and exploit the unique features of cellular systems in under-served communities. Second, *CellChek* accommodates multi-modal sensors, whether mobile phone built-in or on-body medical devices in a seamless manner. Third, we explore cost effective data dissemination that leverages proximity and ubiquity of co-located mobile phones to minimize the cost of data transfer, subject to delay constraints, via sending notifications to a subset of users and leveraging short-range free communication, such as Bluetooth and WiFi, to disseminate information to nearby users.

1.3. Chapter Organization

This chapter is organized as follows. In Section 2, we survey the mobile healthcare literature. Afterwards, Section 3 presents the background and motivation underlying the emerging research area of cost-effective mobile healthcare. The potential benefits of mHealth to under-served communities worldwide, e.g., the elderly community, are highlighted and discussed in Section 4. The focus topic in this chapter, namely cost-effective data transfer from/to a remote patient is presented in Section 5. A proof-of-concept testbed for cost-effective data transfer, coined *CellChek*, is presented in Section 6. Finally, the chapter summary and potential directions for future research are pointed out in Section 7.

2. Mobile Healthcare: Status Quo

The idea of utilizing mobile phones (or PDAs) for remote healthcare systems has gained momentum due to its potential for enhancing the quality of life and reducing the load on the healthcare system [3–12]. However, only recently has the cost aspect come to focus due to its direct relevance to under-served communities and impact on the much needed scalability of mobile healthcare services beyond pilot systems.

In [3], the authors survey recent efforts in this growing area and touch upon proposed standards, architectures and protocols. The smart home care concept and architecture have been introduced in [4]. However, the cost, among other trade-offs, associated with data transfer in under-served communities was out of their scope. The prime focus of [5] has been on energy optimization of Bluetooth-based phone-centered body sensor networks. The work in [6] discusses implementation issues and describes a prototype sensor network for health monitoring using commercial off-the-shelf (COTS) technologies, e.g., IEEE 802.15.4 and custom-built motion and heart activity sensors (e.g., ECG). However, it does not leverage any mobile phone built-in sensors. The CodeBlue project [13] uses a number of medical devices, e.g., pulse oximeter and ECG, that are connected to Zigbee-enabled transmitters. Patients' sensors publish all relevant information while physicians subscribe to the network via multicasting. Physicians can specify the information needed, such as the identification of the patient(s) of interest, and the types of vital signs they need to monitor. Similarly, ALARM-NET [14] provides pervasive and adaptive healthcare for continuous monitoring using environmental and wearable sensors. Care providers may monitor resident health and activity patterns, such as circadian rhythm changes. This frees healthcare practitioners from committing to 24/7 physical monitoring, thus reducing labor costs and increasing efficiency.

On the other hand, [7] exploits the smart phone built-in accelerometer, for elderly activity monitoring. Similarly, when a person accidentally falls, the body part that experiences the initial impact is probably the most affected. In [15], sensors distributed over the body transmit positions through radio devices to a computer, which issues a warning when an accident happens. The system adaptively analyzes body posture and determine the level of injury to provide relevant data to the medical personnel for rescue and treatment.

SMART [16] targets patients in the waiting areas of emergency departments. It has been found that the patient's health deteriorates rapidly while waiting in an emergency room. SMART collects data from various patients waiting in the emergency room and analyzes the data to issue an alert if the health of a particular patient deteriorates.

DexterNet is an open platform, based on the IEEE 802.15.4 standard, for interconnecting on-body medical devices, which has been introduced recently in [9]. However, the trade-offs associated with the wireless Internet connectivity were not addressed. CareNet [17] provides an integrated wireless environment for remote healthcare systems with focus on high reliability and performance, scalability, security and integration with web-based portal systems. In [11], the authors presented a remote tele-presence tele-care system that is based on using robots for monitoring and helping people with special needs. *CellChek* depends on using low-cost ubiquitous mobile phones for achieving the tele-care functionality. The work in [12] presents a smart-home system for monitoring the behavior of diabetes patients and providing ways for altering the incorrect behavior.

On another direction, AID-N [18], the authors target dealing with mass casualty incidents. They use a mesh structure for communication among its different nodes. Patients and medical staff can recognize the correct emergency route through special lights on the AID-N routers.

In 2004, three research initiatives were launched in Egypt towards realizing the e-Health vision [19], namely establishing a Health Record Network (HRN), developing data mining and modeling techniques to better understand the hidden factors contributing to the widespread of certain diseases, and finally developing techniques towards the early detection of breast cancer.

In this chapter, we target an extensible wireless communications system that not only utilizes access technologies, opportunistically, but also accommodates mobile phone built-in sensors as well as on-body medical devices, e.g., Pulse Oximeter and Blood Pressure. In addition, we leverage the proximity and ubiquity of mobile phones to minimize the cost of disseminating public medical data and public health advisories by sending notifications to a subset of the targeted users and utilizing short-range free communication, such as Bluetooth and WiFi, to disseminate information to nearby users. Finally, none of the systems proposed in the literature targets healthcare systems in developing countries and/or under-served communities. This brings about a plethora of new research challenges attributed to pricing (i.e. data plan vs. SMS vs. the dominant pre-paid plans), the limited availability of free public WiFi access and low-income communities. For instance, choosing the optimal (i.e. minimum cost to the user) wireless access technology is an open question for such systems depending on the pricing of the data plan and SMS services, size and type of the data (text, image, video), availability of public vs. subscription-only WiFi. In addition, sending advisory messages from the healthcare provider (HCP) to patients of interest depending on their GPS locations, in a cost- and resource-effective manner, is another research direction presented in this chapter.

3.   Background

3.1.   The Need

Remote healthcare (e-health) is envisioned to have significant impact on the welfare of people, in general, and on the under-served elderly community, in particular. With the continuous advances in healthcare, drug discovery, and quality of life, the number of elderly citizens has been increasing rapidly. In addition, with the continuous pressure of daily life, it is becoming more common for elderly people to live alone for extended periods of time during the day and throughout the year. The World Health Organization (WHO) indicates that the worldwide population of elderly people aged 60 and over are expected to more than double by 2025, and more than triple by 2050 [20]. Moreover, another study shows that over 600 million people worldwide have chronic diseases and over 500 million suffer from aging. In developing countries, where 80% of older people live, the proportion of those over 60 years old in 2025 will increase from 7% to 12%. Moreover, life expectancy at birth has increased globally from 48 years in 1955 to 65 in 1995, and is projected to reach 73 in 2025 [21]. By 2050, people over 80 years old are expected to account for 4% of world's population, up from 1% today [22, 23].

This highlights the strong need for continuous (24/7) medical monitoring which is further aggravated by the fact that qualified healthcare services in under-served communities is either costly or not immediately available. Hence, the "cost" of service comes immediately to the forefront of the problem at hand giving rise to the emerging notion of *cost-effective mobile healthcare*, and associated trade-offs, under investigation in this chapter. This is achieved by using standard mobile phones, localized group communications, and optimally utilizing the wireless communication interfaces depending on the available wireless connectivity, pricing of various services (i.e. data plan, SMS, pre-paid plan), and size and modality of the data. Cost-effective mobile healthcare is also projected to ease the load on the public health system for an important and precious age group that bears the experience, history and culture of any nation represented by the elderly citizens.

3.2. The Opportunity

Mobile phones have achieved significant penetration worldwide over the past decade. At the end of 2010, the International Telecommunication Union (ITU) estimates that there were 5.3 billion mobile subscribers worldwide, including 3.8 billion in developing countries [2]. Access to a mobile network is now available to 90% of the world's population, including 80% of the population living in rural areas. The growth rate in mobile penetration was fastest in sub-saharan Africa, where it grew from less than 2% to 36% between 2000 and 2008, according to ITU statistics [24]. Similar trends hold for the Middle East and North Africa (MENA) region according to Gallup Polls. For instance, Egypt witnessed 64% mobile phone penetration, as opposed to only 9% fixed Internet access penetration, as of Feb. 2009.

Mobile devices are making a significant impact on users worldwide, especially those most vulnerable and geographically hard to reach. The use of mobile devices is transforming the lives of many low-income communities, by giving people access to health information, eliminating the cost of transportation to access services, among other benefits.

From the perspective of features, sensors and supported applications, mobile phones can be roughly categorized to:

- *Basic phones:* support core functionalities, e.g., voice, SMS messaging.

- *Internet-enabled Phones:* support, beyond the core capabilities, Internet access for sending e-mails, browsing the web, etc.

- *Smart phones:* support, beyond the Internet-enabled phones, a wide range of sensors, e.g., GPS, accelerometer, ambient light, and camera) and a plethora of applications.

The importance of the above characterization stems from the following key observations: i) The mobile phones used in low income communities are predominantly basic phones, ii) Internet-enabled phones penetration is rapidly increasing within the middle class and iii) Smart phones are the only sensor-rich phones, enabling a wide variety of innovative applications using these sensors, e.g., the accelerometer (for fall detection [25]). Thus, it is straightforward to distill the following conclusions. First, SMS messaging will play a key role in mHealth, in general, and in cost-effective mHealth in particular due to its low cost and guaranteed support on every mobile phone in the market. Thus, we give SMS special attention in the interface selection algorithm on the uplink as well as the cost-delay trade-off on the downlink. Second, even though wireless data services are available today on all smart phones and most Internet-enabled phones, they may not be available on all basic phones. However, the witnessed price trends for consumer electronics over the past decade (thanks to Moore's Law) project that the Internet-enabled phones should be affordable to low income communities in the near future and smart phones should follow few years after. Thus, we embrace this projection in the chapter and consider sensor-rich smart phones, with multiple wireless interfaces, under the assumption of being affordable across the board in the future. Third, data plans in low-income communities are predominantly of the pre-paid type. Unlimited data plans are not of great interest in our "cost-effective" context since they are neither affordable nor needed by disadvantaged communities targeted in our study.

In conclusion, the rapid growth of mobile phone penetration, complemented by a plethora of wireless standards and new use cases (e.g., mCommerce, Learning and Health), has inspired novel applications that range from social to business. This creates an ample opportunity for the cost-effective mHealth paradigm which lies at the intersection of disparate research areas, namely mobile communications and healthcare for under-served communities where remote healthcare is mostly needed.

4. Benefits to Under-served Communities

Cost-effective mobile healthcare is expected to have significant impact on the health of the society in general and the under-served elderly community in particular. With the continuous advances in healthcare, drug discovery, and quality of life, the number of elderly citizens has been increasing rapidly. In addition, with the continuous pressure of daily life, it is becoming more common for elderly people to be living alone for extended periods of time during the day and throughout the year. Despite the fact that the Egyptian government considers elderly care as one of the most fundamental human issues that receives the state's due attention [26], the number of elderly homes in 2006 of 104, benefiting about 2400 senior citizens, is far from covering the millions of Egyptians whose age is above 65 years [27]. The percentage of the elderly in the population has been steadily increasing according to the general census of the population in Egypt [20, 28] reaching 5.1% in 1950 and up to 6.3% in 2000. It is projected to increase to 11.5% in 2025 and further reach up to 20.8% in 2050. This highlights the pressing need for Information and Communications Technology (ICT) help to improve the effectiveness and timeliness of healthcare services offered to this important sector of the Egyptian society. In 1996, the census shows that majority of the elderly in Egypt are in the age group 60-64 years and constitute 41% of the overall ratio of the elderly, followed by the age group of 65-70 years (27%), followed by the age group 70+ years (32%).

To close this gap and to provide support for the increasing number of elderly citizens who live alone, mobile healthcare aims at providing ubiquitous healthcare, based on the use of the widespread sensor-rich mobile phones along with emerging wireless-enabled medical devices. The system is capable of sending patient reminders, including "Time for Medication", detecting emergency situations, and periodic checks, among other services.

Emergency situations such as sudden falling, strokes, heart attacks, and long periods of inactivity, can be detected by gathering and transferring sensor data from the elderly citizens in a timely manner. This data can be processed on the mobile phone, to generate alerts, or sent directly to the medical personnel for 24/7 monitoring and analysis.

The cost-effective mobile healthcare paradigm will address problems related to sensors integration and communication. In particular, we address the problems of leveraging built-in phones sensors and attaching portable non-intrusive medical devices to the elderly person to remotely monitor vital signs, such as heart pulse rate, ECG, and motion. Relaying the data and/or alerts to interested parties using the available communication channels is another direction for this work.

Such system is expected to have a significant impact on the healthcare services offered to the elderly, not only in Egypt, but also throughout the region and internationally. It is expected that the system will reduce the load on the public health system for an important and precious age group that bears the experience, history and culture of any nation represented by the elderly citizens.

5. Cost-effective Networking: A New Paradigm for mHealth

In this section, we introduce the novel concept of cost-effective mobile health-care with particular emphasis on data transfer to/from a remote patient, e.g., periodic checkups for chronic diseases. This should contribute to major cost savings manifested in saving the transportation cost to/from the healthcare facility in addition to saving the medical team time and effort for more urgent causes.

5.1. Cost-effective Medical Data Upload

In this section, we focus on uploading the patient's gathered medical data, using the mobile phone, with minimum cost, in an attempt to save costs to individuals. Towards this objective, we introduce a lightweight wireless interface selection algorithm (WISA), running on the mobile phone, to decide the "optimal" radio interface (from a cost saving perspective).

5.1.1. The Wireless Interface Selection Algorithm (WISA)

The WISA algorithm decides the minimum cost wireless interface subject to the available connectivity options, data size, modality and QoS (particularly delay) constraints. In essence, the WISA algorithm, outlined in Figure 1, checks the availability of public (free) WiFi access, Bluetooth peer-to-peer (p2p) connectivity, and cellular 3G in this order, due to the zero-cost advantage of the former two connectivity options. Thus, at the first step, WISA searches for free opportunistic WiFi. If not found, the p2p mode is activated (Bluetooth/WiFi) to check for a nearby mobile phone (namely gateway) connected to the Internet and willing to upload the data. It is worth noting that the p2p mode is explored as a fundamental concept in this chapter whereas quantifying its cost benefits

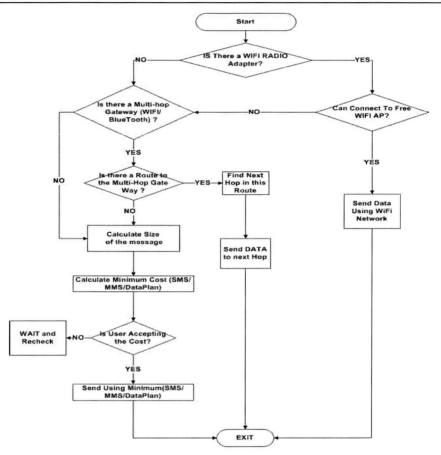

Figure 1. The Wireless Interface Selection Algorithm (WISA).

and potential trade-offs lie out of the scope of this work and is a subject of future research. Otherwise, WISA concludes that there is no free wireless option and, hence, the non-zero cost 3G options need to be explored next. Accordingly, WISA computes the data size and depending on the its type (i.e. plain text, image, video) decides the minimum cost 3G transport protocol to be used, namely data plan, short message service (SMS) or multimedia message service (MMS). Finally, if the previous options are not available, WISA enters into a waiting mode and retries again depending on the delay tolerance of the application. If the data is time-sensitive, the user is alerted to purchase the minimum amount of credit or urged to accept the minimum cost.

Next, we present the data transfer accounting as a major building block of WISA. *A. Data Transfer Accounting:* In order to decide the minimum cost cellular data transfer protocol, the cost of sending the data using the data plan needs to be quantified. On one hand, the cost of sending a single SMS (or MMS) is constant as specified by the cellular operator. If the data size exceeds the maximum SMS (or MMS) size, then the incurred cost is linearly proportional to the number of messages needed. On the other hand, quantifying the cost using a limited data plan is less trivial. Towards this objective, we surveyed various data plans offered by Egypt's major cellular operators. As a representative of limited data plans (of interest to low-income communities), we assume a generic time-limited plan with a pre-specified quota (in MBytes) available for use. If the quota is exceeded, the user is charged at a higher rate for each extra byte. Accordingly, there are two key observations pertaining to this type of plans,

1. In case of utilizing a small percentage of the available quota (i.e. under utilization), the user is charged for the entire cost of the plan, which implies that per byte price will be higher compared to the case where the plan is fully utilized.

2. In case of utilizing extra Mega Bytes (MB) beyond the plan's pre-specified quota (i.e. over utilization), the user is charged at a very high rate per extra byte compared to the rate-per-byte within the limited quota.

Next, we derive the cost per Mega Byte for the considered time-limited data-plan under two cases. First, when the data plan usage has not exceeded the pre-specified quota. Second, when the plan usage exceeds the quota, an additional term would be needed in order to account for the price of the beyond-quota usage. In both cases, the cost of one MB is calculated as the payment by the end of the plan divided by the expected number of MBs used throughout the plan duration.

Towards the above stated objectives, we introduce the following system model and appropriate notation. We consider a single medical event that takes place at an instant of time where t hours remain until the data plan expires and n MB until the quota is consumed. This medical event generates data of size Z MB. We model non-medical data plan usage events as a constant bit rate (CBR) process with rate L (MB/hr). It is worth noting that these events are independent of the single medical event at hand. The data plan time limit is denoted T hours and its limited quota is assumed to be A MB. Finally, the price of the limited-quota data plan is P Egyptian Pounds (EGP) and the price per extra MB is p EGP.

Case I: If the expected plan usage, upon expiry, does not exceed the quota limit, i.e. $((A-n)+Z+L*t) \leq A$, then the cost per MB would be given by,

$$Cost_{MB} = \frac{P}{((A-n)+Z+L*t)} \tag{1}$$

Case II: If the expected plan usage, upon expiry, exceeds the quota limit, i.e. $((A-n)+Z+L*t) > A$, then the cost per MB would include an additional term to account for the beyond-the-quota usage,

$$Cost_{MB} = \frac{(P+p*(Z+L*t-n))}{((A-n)+Z+L*t)} \tag{2}$$

Hence, the cost of uploading the Z MBs generated by the medical event is given by,

$$Cost_Z = Cost_{MB} * Z \tag{3}$$

Towards the results in (1.1) and (1.2), we first calculate the expected data usage (in MBs), by the plan expiry date and time, as follows,

$$Expected\ Usage = ((A-n)+Z+L*t) \tag{4}$$

where $(A-n)$ is the number of MBs consumed upon the medical event occurrence, Z is the medical event size, and $L*t$ is the number of non-medical MB usage until data plan expiry. If the expected usage does not exceed the data plan quota, i.e. $((A-n)+Z+L*t) \leq A$, then the result in (1.1) can be directly derived by dividing the plan cost, P, by (1.4).

On the other hand, if the expected usage exceeds the data plan quota, i.e. $((A-n)+Z+L*t) > A$, then we should account for the extra MBs cost. This is achieved via subtracting the quota from the total usage of the plan as given by,

$$Extra\ Usage = ((A-n)+Z+L*t) - A \tag{5}$$

Thus, the MB cost in this case is calculated as the summation of the limited quota MB cost and *Extra Usage* MB cost as given in (1.2).

Equation (1.3) shows the MB cost trends with the variables t and n for the above two cases as demonstrated in Figure 2. It shows that the MB cost has the two extreme cases discussed before; when the plan usage is very low compared to the quota (i.e. $n << A$), this implies high MB cost. On the other hand, when the quota is exceeded, the MB cost becomes very high due to the higher cost p per MB.

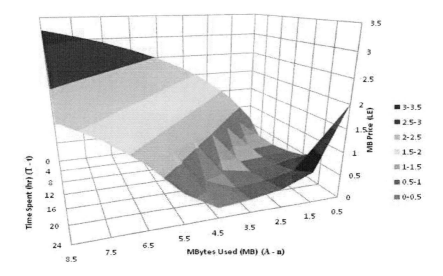

Figure 2. Data Plan Mega Byte Cost.

As a major component of WISA, the trends in Figure 2 provide valuable insights to assess the viability of using the data plan as opposed to other options such as SMS or MMS.

5.1.2. Scenarios Illustrating WISA Operation

1. **Scenario I:** Data Upload using WiFi

   (a) If a free Wi-Fi Access Point (AP) is available.

(b) If the mobile phone is already connected to a WiFi AP for other purposes, even if not free. WiFi can be leveraged as free from the WISA perspective since its already connected.

2. **Scenario II:** Data Upload using SMS

If free WiFi is not available and the data is low size plain text that can be sent using SMS with cost less than the data plan. Next, we provide an exemplary scenario for illustration.

Example 1:
Gathered medical data size (Z) = 50 Bytes.
Time limit of the data plan (T) = 24 hours (1 day).
Data plan quota (A) = 5 MB.
Price of the data plan (P) = 1 EGP.
Price of an extra MB (p)= 5 EGP.
Assume t corresponds to 18 hours remining in the plan, i.e. $t = 18$.
Assume no data plan usage, other than medical (i.e. L=0).
Assume the MBs remaining until the plan quota is consumed, n = 5 MB, i.e. nothing used yet.
WISA Decision:
Cost of data plan computed using (1.3) = 1 EGP.
Cost of SMS = 0.3 EGP.
Decision: Upload data using SMS.

3. **Scenario III:** Data Upload using 3G/GPRS Data Plan

If free WiFi is not available, the data is of any type and size and the cost of the data plan is less than SMS/MMS. This is illustrated via the following example.

Example 2:
Gathered medical data size (Z) = 50 Bytes.
Assume a fixed rate of non-medical data plan usage, L=0.1 MB/hour.
Time limit of the data plan (T) = 24 hours (1 day).
Data plan quota (A) = 5 MB.
Price of the data plan (P) = 1 EGP.
Price of an extra MB (p) = 5 EGP.

Assume t corresponds to 18 hours remining in the plan.

Assume the MBs remaining until the plan quota is consumed, $n = 4$ MB.

WISA Decision:

Cost of data plan computed using (1.3) < 0.01 EGP (since only at the 6th hour the user still has most of the quota, 4 MB).

Cost of SMS = 0.3 EGP.

Decision: Upload data using data plan.

5.2. Cost-effective Advisory Message Dissemination

In this section, we shift our attention to the cost-effective medical, or generally public, advisory message (e.g., SMS) dissemination on the downlink, i.e. from the healthcare provider (HCP) server to a "co-located" target group of patients or senior citizens in a senior housing facility. The concept underlying the sought cost savings in this setting hinges on the novel idea of leveraging the readily available *free* phone-to-phone communication wireless interface (e.g., Bluetooth or WiFi operating in the Ad hoc mode) in order to disseminate the messages in a multi-hop fashion to cover the target group. Our ultimate goal is to provide cost-effective downlink data dissemination to the users subject to application delay constraints.

5.2.1. Problem Statement

Consider the problem of disseminating a single advisory message, say by the local health authority, to a group of M target users.[1] The straightforward approach towards accomplishing this task is via sending M messages (possibly SMS), one directed to each user. Hence, the cost incurred would grow linearly with the size of the target group M which would be a limit, especially for developing countries, when the size of the group scales. In an attempt to circumvent this linear growth hurdle, the approach proposed in this chapter is two phase: i) *Phase 1:* The HCP server disseminates the target message to a subset of strategically located users (called hubs) and ii) *Phase 2:* the hubs take the burden of disseminating the message further to the rest $(M - N)$ users, essentially forming an ad hoc network. Despite the simplicity of the idea, it gives rise to interesting

---

[1]We assume in this chapter that the target users are geographically co-located. However, this assumption can be relaxed based on the ubiquity and wide spread of mobile phones worldwide.

Cost-QoS trade-offs, particularly a cost-delay trade-off which we will highlight in the next section.

5.2.2. The Cost-Delay Trade-off

In this section, we characterize the cost-delay trade-off pertaining to the problem of efficient message dissemination from the HCP server to remote co-located mobile phones. We develop a simple theoretical model for the mobile phone ad hoc network that adequately captures the cost-delay trade-off and its related dynamics. We consider M stationary nodes uniformly distributed over a circular region of radius R. All nodes have equal transmission ranges, denoted r. Asymptotically (i.e. as $M \to \infty$), the circular region can be approximately divided into N circular sub-regions (also called clusters) where the N mobile phone hubs are assumed to reside at the centers of those sub-regions and would be responsible for disseminating to members of its respective sub-regions. Thus, the area of each cluster would scale as $O(\pi R^2/N)$ and, hence, the radius of an arbitrary cluster, denoted R_c, scales as $O(R/\sqrt{N})$. Based on the fixed transmission range assumption for each node, it is straightforward to conclude that the average number of hops to propagate data within a cluster is $O(R/(\sqrt{N} * r))$ which is the radius of the cluster divided by the node's transmission range r. In order to simplify the model and capture the crux of the problem, we assume the presence of a perfect MAC protocol that coordinates nodes transmissions and completely eliminates interference. Thus, we do not account for MAC delays in our model since it is expected to affect the exact values for link delays but not the fundamental trade-off at hand.

Based on the above discussion, quantifying the cost associated with sending N messages, $C(N)$, is simply a linear function of the cost of single message, denoted S, that is, $C(N) = N * S$. On the other hand, quantifying the end-to-end (E2E) delay, D_{E2E}, defined as the time elapsed between sending the message at the HCP server until it reaches all M nodes, turned out to be more involved. At the outset, the E2E delay is simply the summation of the delay in Phase 1 and the delay in Phase 2. The delay incurred in Phase 1 is relatively simple as it essentially amounts to the average message delay from the HCP server to all mobile phone hubs, denoted D_{3G}, assuming transmission to the N mobile phone hubs takes place exactly in parallel. As for Phase 2, the delay involved while forwarding a message from a hub to its cluster members, denoted D_{manet}, is quantified as follows. First, it is straightforward to notice that the worst-case ad hoc network delay is given by the product of the average phone-to-phone link delay and the maximum number of hops to cover the cluster (i.e. the cluster radius quantified above), that is,

$$D_{manet} = D_l * R_c \qquad (6)$$

where D_l is the average link delay and R_c is the cluster radius. Second, the wireless link delay is known to accommodate the average transmission delay (D_t), average queuing delay (D_q), propagation delay (D_p), processing delay ($D_p r$) and average MAC delay (D_{MAC}). In our system, we ignore the propagation delays due to the short distances traveled (order of meters) in case of co-located mobile phones, the processing delays thanks to Moore's law and, finally, the MAC delays assuming the presence of an ideal zero-delay MAC. Therefore, the link delay amounts to,

$$D_l = D_t + D_q \qquad (7)$$

where,

$$D_t = \frac{Z}{B} \qquad (8)$$

where Z is the message size (in bits) and B is the p2p link bit rate (in bps) and,

$$D_q = \frac{\rho}{2\mu(1-\rho)} \qquad (9)$$

based on an M/D/1 queuing model [29], where $\rho = \lambda * D_t$ is the system loading factor and λ is the rate of arrival of transmission requests to the queue of the phone-to-phone wireless interface, assumed to be Poisson in our model and D_t is the average service (message transmission) time. Therefore, the end-to-end delay denoted as D_{E2E} is given by,

$$D_{E2E} = D_{3G} + D_{manet} \qquad (10)$$

Given the above model, it is evident that decreasing the number of mobile phone hubs, N, reduces the cost, yet, at the expense of longer delays in Phase 2. Notice that Phase 1 delay is always constant and always present for any choice of N. In fact, Phase 1 delay constitutes the lower bound on the E2E delay achievable only in the extreme case of $N = M$, i.e. there is essentially no Phase 2. Thus, the quest for the optimal number of gateways that strikes a balance between minimizing cost and minimizing E2E delays can be formulated as a constrained optimization problem for minimizing the cost subject to a delay requirement, denoted x, that is,

$$min_N C(N) \tag{11}$$

$$s.t. \, D_{E2E} \leq x$$

Fortunately, this problem can solved in closed form using Lagrange multipliers [30],

$$g(N,\gamma) = C(N) + \gamma(D_{E2E} - x) \tag{12}$$

where γ is the Lagrange multiplier. By differentiating with respect to N and equating to zero,

$$\frac{\partial g}{\partial N} = 0$$

we get optimal N as a function of γ,

$$N^* = [\frac{\gamma * R * D_{manet}}{2 * S * r}]^{\frac{2}{3}} \tag{13}$$

and we get γ through the constraint $D_{E2E} = x$

$$\gamma^{\frac{1}{3}} = \frac{(2 * S)^{1/3}(R * D_{manet})^{2/3}}{r^{2/3}(x - D_{3G})} \tag{14}$$

So the optimal number of mobile phone hubs N is ,

$$N^* = [\frac{R * D_{manet}}{r\,(x - D_{3G})}]^2 \tag{15}$$

According to (15), the optimal number of mobile phone hubs, N^*, is independent of the message 3G transmission cost S which may seem counterintuitive at a first glance. However, this result turns out to agree with intuition due to the linear dependence of the communication cost on S, that is, $C(N) = N * S$. Thus, minimizing the message dissemination cost subject to the delay constraint x, yields a minimum (optimal) number of hubs N below which the delay requirement, x, would be violated. The optimal, N^*, is independent of S which only affects the slope of the linear cost function and, hence, the cost-delay intersection point when plotted versus N as shown in Figure 3 . However, the intersection point constitutes the optimal (that minimizes both cost and delay) which is different from the constrained optimization problem at hand in (11) which is primarily driven by the delay constraint, x.

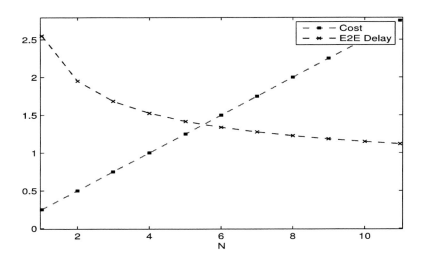

Figure 3. Dissemination cost and E2E delay trends vs. the Number of hubs, N.

5.2.3.   Numerical Results

Using the above model, numerical results are generated to confirm the trade-off and show the optimal N^* for plausible message dissemination scenarios for a group of co-located mobile phones, e.g., in a senior housing facility. This analysis is conducted given the following model parameters: R=5000m, r=50m, S=0.25 EGP, D_t=0.02 sec for Z=5KB message and B=2 Mbps link bit rate, λ =0.1 message per second and $D_{3G} = 0.5$ sec. Finally, it can be shown that D_q=2.1015e-05.

Next, we present numerical results that not only confirm the cost-delay trade-off but also quantifies the optimal number of mobile phone hubs, N^*, as we change the delay constraint, x, from delay-sensitive to delay-tolerant applications.

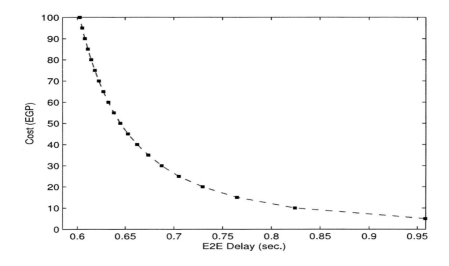

Figure 4. Communication cost-Delay trade-off.

As shown in Figure 4, the total message dissemination cost is plotted against the E2E delay which confirms the fundamental trade-off. Each point on the curve corresponds to a value of N that yields the certain cost and delay. The figure shows that as the number of hubs N increases, the cost increases, yet, the E2E delay decreases. The optimum N is the value that obtains the minimum cost subject to the pre-specified delay threshold, x.

On the other hand, Figure 5 quantifies the optimal number of mobile phone hubs, N^*, as a function of x. As the delay tolerance increases, the system allows more hops to reach destinations in an attempt to reduce the cost. Hence, the number of mobile phone hubs needed to disseminate the message can be reduced as shown from the given trend.

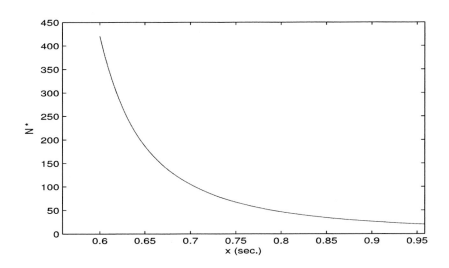

Figure 5. Optimum number of hubs N^* versus different delay thresholds, x.

6. The *CellChek* Testbed

6.1. The Overall Architecture

The *CellChek* system (shown in Figure 6) accommodates two types of sensors. First, external Bluetooth-enabled medical devices such as blood pressure monitor and pulse oximeter. Second, mobile phone built-in sensors (e.g., accelerometer , GPS and camera). As shown in Figure 7, the mobile phone collects the sensory data and transmits it to the HCP server through two stages. First, the patient directs the *CellChek* mobile software to read the measurements from the on-body medical devices and the mobile phone built-in sensors as shown in Figure 7(a). Second, the patient uploads the data through SMS/MMS or the Internet (WiFi/3G data plan) in a cost-effective manner using the WISA algorithm as shown in Figure 7(b). Care givers can access the HCP server anytime via a web interface to remotely monitor their patients.

Moreover, as shown in Figure 6, *CellChek* provides a cost-effective advisory dissemination service via sending notifications to a subset of the target mobile phones from the HCP server and utilizing the short-range free phone-to-phone

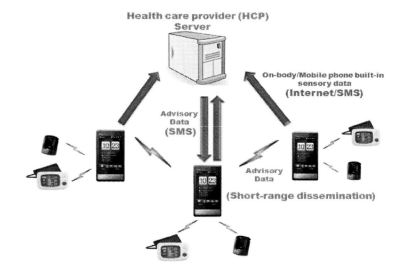

Figure 6. *CellChek* Overall Architecture.

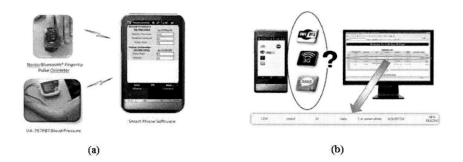

Figure 7. *CellChek* System Operation: a) Sensor data collection and b) Transmitting sensor data through the most cost-effective interface to the HCP server where care givers monitor their patients through a web interface.

communication capability, such as WiFi and Bluetooth, to disseminate information to nearby mobile phones.

In the remaining of this section, we overview the Bluetooth-enabled medical devices used in *CellChek* and present exemplary use cases that not only showcase the system in operation but also demonstrate its utility for supporting healthcare services on the move as well as for elderly citizens living alone.

6.2.   Medical Devices

The *CellChek* system leverages two major types of sensors, namely Bluetooth-enabled on-body medical devices and mobile phone built-in sensors. Next, we review these devices and their main features and capabilities demonstrated in *CellChek*.

- On-body Bluetooth-enabled Medical Devices

  We use a Bluetooth fingertip pulse oximeter from Nonin (Nonin Onyx II Model 9560 Bluetooth Fingertip Pulse Oximeter) [31]. This device is chosen due to its track record in prior research as well as its ability to provide reasonably reliable measurements for oxygen saturation range (Spo2) and pulse rate range (beats per minute).

  In addition, we use a Bluetooth-enabled blood pressure monitor from A&D Medical (UA-767PBT Blood Pressure Monitoring device A&D) [32] which provides blood pressure (systolic pressure and diastolic pressure) and pulse rate measurements. Blood pressure regular monitoring is essential for patients as well as high-risk elderly citizens with chronic diseases.

  Measurements are collected from the above medical devices(shown in Figure 8) using a Bluetooth connection between the mobile phone and the medical device.

- Mobile Phone Built-in Sensors

  Accelerometer (*GSensor*) have been used in the literature for a variety of applications, e.g. for medical purposes to monitor the activity of the owner. In our system, the accelerometer has been exploited for fall detection. The basic algorithm for fall detection relies on the magnitude

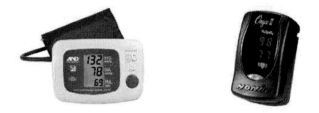

Figure 8. Bluetooth-enabled Blood Pressure Monitor from A&D (left) and Fingertip Pulse Oximeter from Nonin (right).

value of the components of the accelerometer readings [25]. Using the accelerometer onboard on most smart phone available today, access to the accelerometer readings is attained through the manufacturer's SDK. Thanks to the evolution in mobile software development we are able to access the accelerometer readings from C# (.NET) code. The magnitude of the accelerometer reading is measured in meters per second squared. Ideally, when the device is in a motionless state, the vector would be of length 9.8 (the gravitational constant). However, the sensor is not extremely accurate, so this is almost never the case. This magnitude changes with different motions such that in the case of falling there is an acceleration component added to the original magnitude of the accelerometer reading, and, hence, a fall can be easily detected [25].

GPS can be used to specify the patient location in case of emergency conditions. The GPS readings can be revealed by the SDK presented with most mobile phone manufacturers to access their GPS devices for use in numerous location-based services emerging on most smart phones today.

6.3.   Example Use Cases

In this section, we present exemplary use cases for the *CellChek* system that not only showcase the system in operation but also demonstrate its utility for supporting healthcare services on the move as well as for elderly citizens living alone.

6.3.1. Use Case 1: Monitoring a Patient on the Move

Consider a passenger riding a vehicle/bus/metro who needs to be continuously monitored for sudden abnormal conditions. The passenger wouldn't be worried for his health, while practicing his normal life activities, as long as he is remotely monitored by *CellChek*, at minimum cost. The system can be easily started by connecting the wireless medical devices to the patient's body and allowing the *CellChek* mobile software to read the measurements from the on-body medical devices. *CellChek* generates a medical profile that contains the patient's measurements. Afterwards, the gathered data is uploaded to the HCP server using the WISA algorithm which chooses the most cost effective wireless interface available.

The HCP server receives the medical profile and saves it in the appropriate database. The user medical profile can be shown on the *CellChek* website which can be monitored by the care givers anywhere, anytime. The system can also be used to monitor the states of the patients 24/7, fire alarms and send advisory messages, if needed.

6.3.2. Use Case 2: Fall Detection and Reporting

CellChek communicates with the mobile phone built-in sensor, namely the accelerometer, via accessing the driver of the device on the mobile phone. The accelerometer main usage is to monitor falling conditions, it raises an alarm to the mobile user in case of fall detection. If the user does not respond to the alarm (indicating an emergency situation), the system automatically generates a medical profile that describes the patient's situation and sends the data directly to the HCP server. If it is impossible to reach the server (due to lack of Internet connectivity), then it sends the alarm via SMS to a predefined emergency number.

The HCP server receives the medical profile with a specific medical record number and saves it on the subscribed patient record in the database, using the patient's medical record number.

Care givers can detect falling conditions through the *CellChek* website. This web-server is the central point for the data gathered from all subscribers in the system and can be used to monitor the states of the patients continuously, fire alarms, and sending advisory information when needed.

7. Summary

In this chapter, we presented a new research paradigm in the emerging mobile healthcare research arena, namely cost-effective data transfer, targeted towards bringing qualified medical attention to under-served communities at minimum cost as well as potentially saving major expenses to healthcare authorities and insurance companies worldwide. The problem of providing qualified and timely medical attention to under-served communities around the world, and in developing countries in particular, has been a major challenge for the international community, at least for the last decade. This problem is further aggravated by the fact that healthcare services are either too costly or not immediately available in those parts of the world.

On the other hand, and over the same period of time, the ICT domain has been witnessing a number of major developments independently. First, the convergence of sensing and actuation, communications and computing constitutes the key enabler for a multitude of miniaturized and embedded platforms and devices around us, giving rise to a "connected-world", be it in the environment, at home, workplace, industrial plants or even in the human body for treatment and remote monitoring purposes. Second, the wireless technology wide proliferation has inspired many novel applications and services that range from social, business, national security, and defense to education and healthcare-related services. Third, the continuous increase of the number of mobile subscribers around the world and the developing world, as confirmed by recent ITU reports and estimates, creates ample opportunity for ubiquitous (i.e. anywhere, anytime) services.

The novel marriage of the need for healthcare services for low-income communities and the prevailing opportunity presented by the wide proliferation of Internet-capable mobile phones sets the perfect stage for a new research paradigm which constitutes the subject matter of this chapter, namely cost-effective mobile healthcare. Mobile healthcare is a rapidly growing multidisciplinary research area as evidenced by recent diverse literature from the wireless communications, sensor networking, mobile computing, and medical communities. Nevertheless, the emphasis on cost savings as a major design driver, rather than after-the-fact issue, is still in its infancy and has not received sufficient attention from the community.

In this chapter, we introduced this ripe area of research and shed some light on a specific problem within this space, namely cost-effective data transfer via leveraging the multiple radio interfaces available on smart phones today, and soon will be available on a wide range of mobile phones, including low-end phones, thanks to the Very Large Scale Integration (VLSI) industry trends projected by Moore's law. The envisioned cost-effective mobile healthcare system, coined *CellChek*, is not only optimized to overcome a unique set of challenges inherent to mobile phone usage in low-income communities (e.g., expensive data plans, predominantly pre-paid plans, limited public WiFi access) but also poised to effectively exploit a unique set of features inherent to Cellular 3G systems (e.g., free incoming calls, inexpensive SMS service). *CellChek* is envisioned to leverage a plethora of sensing modalities ranging from wireless-enabled on-body medical devices (e.g., blood pressure, pulse oximeter and ECG) to mobile phone built-in sensors (e.g., accelerometer, GPS and camera).

Towards the aforementioned objectives, we presented *CellChek* as a proof-of-concept testbed for cost-effective ubiquitous mobile healthcare systems based on the use of sensor-rich mobile phones along with emerging wireless-enabled medical devices. First, we proposed the wireless interface selection algorithm (WISA) which selects the wireless interface that yields minimum cost, depending on the size of the data to be uploaded, its modality (plain text, voice, image, video) and quality of service (QoS), particularly delay, constraints. Second, we developed a theoretical model for the medical advisory message dissemination problem that adequately captures the cost-delay trade-off when leveraging free phone-to-phone communications, possibly using Bluetooth or WiFi. Finally, we presented the major components of *CellChek*, its functional description and demonstrated its operation and benefits with the aid of two use cases, namely leveraging the accelerometer for fall detection and remote patient monitoring. We strongly believe that the concept of cost-effective mobile healthcare presented in this chapter holds a great promise within the mobile healthcare arena and is equally important for developing and developed countries.

7.1. Future Research Directions

With the pressing need for enhanced, timely and reliable medical services and the increasing trends of mobile phone subscribers witnessed around the world, the breadth and depth of the mobile healthcare research portfolio will only continue to increase to cater to the surging demand. Cost-effective mobile healthcare is a ripe area of research that needs further attention from the wireless, networking and mobile computing research communities along the following research thrusts, among many others:

- The concept of "Cost-Effective" mobile healthcare is still in its infancy. In this chapter we touched upon a specific research topic, namely cost effective data transfer. However, this ripe area of research needs further exploration along multiple directions towards the research, design and development of cost-effective on-body sensing platforms (e.g., bluetooth-enabled ECG known to be expensive), cost-effective mobile computing architectures and data storage systems and, finally, balancing the associated design trade-offs with cost.

- Introduce a delay tolerant networking (DTN) architecture as a key enabler for cost-effective mobile healthcare that remains a largely unexplored territory. For instance, exploring the potential trade-offs of opportunistically leveraging free public WiFi access, if the healthcare application delay constraints permit.

- Explore the notion of multi-hop phone-to-phone communications for possibly uploading the medical data via other phones in the neighborhood with Internet access. This novel paradigm gives rise to a number of research challenges, namely cooperation and incentive-based schemes, game-theoretic formulations and patient medical record privacy issues.

- Explore and balance the fundamental security-cost trade-offs attributed to the data size increase contributed by classical security mechanisms. This involves, among other design issues, the development of lightweight security schemes with minimum overhead (cost).

- Integrate ECG devices to the *CellChek* testbed and develop lightweight data compression algorithms, for the immense amount of data generated by ECG, suitable for resource-limited basic and Internet-enabled mobile phones.

References

[1] K. Siau, "Health care informatics," *Information Technology in Biomedicine, IEEE Transactions on*, vol. 7, no. 1, pp. 1–7, 2003.

[2] "The world in 2010: Ict facts and figures," International Telecommunication Union, Tech. Rep., 2010.

[3] A. Kailas and M. Ingram, "Wireless communications technology in tele-health systems," in *Wireless Communication, Vehicular Technology, Information Theory and Aerospace & Electronic Systems Technology, 2009. Wireless VITAE 2009. 1st International Conference on.* IEEE, 2009, pp. 926–930.

[4] P. Leijdekkers, V. Gay, and E. Lawrence, "Smart homecare system for health tele-monitoring," in *Proceedings of the First International Conference on the Digital Society.* Washington, DC, USA: IEEE Computer Society, 2007, p. 3. [Online]. Available: http://portal.acm.org/citation.cfm?id=1260201.1260513

[5] L. Zhong, M. Sinclair, and R. Bittner, "A phone-centered body sensor network platform: cost, energy efficiency & user interface," 2006.

[6] A. Milenkovic, C. Otto, and E. Jovanov, "Wireless sensor networks for personal health monitoring: Issues and an implementation," *Computer Communications*, vol. 29, no. 13-14, pp. 2521–2533, 2006.

[7] Y. Hong, I. Kim, S. Ahn, and H. Kim, "Activity recognition using wearable sensors for elder care," in *Future Generation Communication and Networking, 2008. FGCN'08. Second International Conference on*, vol. 2. IEEE, 2008, pp. 302–305.

[8] A. Prentza, S. Maglavera, and L. Leondaridis, "Delivery of healthcare services over mobile phones: e-vital and chs paradigms," in *Engineering in Medicine and Biology Society, 2006. EMBS'06. 28th Annual International Conference of the IEEE.* IEEE, 2006, pp. 3250–3253.

[9] R. Istepanian and J. Lacal, "Emerging mobile communication technologies for health: some imperative notes on m-health," in *Engineering in*

Medicine and Biology Society, 2003. Proceedings of the 25th Annual International Conference of the IEEE, vol. 2.   IEEE, 2003, pp. 1414–1416.

[10] P. Kuryloski, A. Giani, R. Giannantonio, K. Gilani, R. Gravina, V. Seppa, E. Seto, V. Shia, C. Wang, P. Yan *et al.*, "Dexternet: An open platform for heterogeneous body sensor networks and its applications," in *Wearable and Implantable Body Sensor Networks, 2009. BSN 2009. Sixth International Workshop on.*   IEEE, 2009, pp. 92–97.

[11] A. Helal and B. Abdulrazak, "Tecarob: Tele-care using telepresence and robotic technology for assisting people with special needs," *International Journal of Human-friendly Welfare Robotic Systems*, vol. 7, no. 3, 2006.

[12] A. Helal, D. Cook, and M. Schmalz, "Smart home-based health platform for behavioral monitoring and alteration of diabetes patients," *Journal of diabetes science and technology (Online)*, vol. 3, no. 1, p. 141, 2009.

[13] V. Shnayder, B. Chen, K. Lorincz, T. Fulford-Jones, and M. Welsh, "Sensor networks for medical care," in *SenSys 05: Proceedings of the 3rd international conference on Embedded networked sensor systems.*   Citeseer, 2005, pp. 314–314.

[14] A. Wood, G. Virone, T. Doan, Q. Cao, L. Selavo, Y. Wu, L. Fang, Z. He, S. Lin, and J. Stankovic, "Alarm-net: Wireless sensor networks for assisted-living and residential monitoring," *University of Virginia Computer Science Department Technical Report*, 2006.

[15] C. Lai, Y. Huang, H. Chao, and J. Park, "Adaptive body posture analysis using collaborative multi-sensors for elderly falling detection," *IEEE Intelligent Systems*, 2010.

[16] D. Curtis, E. Shih, J. Waterman, J. Guttag, J. Bailey, T. Stair, R. Greenes, and L. Ohno-Machado, "Physiological signal monitoring in the waiting areas of an emergency room," in *Proceedings of the ICST 3rd international conference on Body area networks.*   ICST (Institute for Computer Sciences, Social-Informatics and Telecommunications Engineering), 2008, pp. 1–8.

[17] S. Jiang, Y. Cao, S. Iyengar, P. Kuryloski, R. Jafari, Y. Xue, R. Bajcsy, and S. Wicker, "Carenet: an integrated wireless sensor networking environment for remote healthcare," in *Proceedings of the ICST 3rd international conference on Body area networks*. ICST (Institute for Computer Sciences, Social-Informatics and Telecommunications Engineering), 2008, p. 9.

[18] T. Gao, T. Massey, L. Selavo, D. Crawford, B. Chen, K. Lorincz, V. Shnayder, L. Hauenstein, F. Dabiri, J. Jeng *et al.*, "The advanced health and disaster aid network: A light-weight wireless medical system for triage," *Biomedical Circuits and Systems, IEEE Transactions on*, vol. 1, no. 3, pp. 203–216, 2007.

[19] "A new era for ict in egypt: R&d promises and challenges," Ministry of Communications and Information Technology, IST 2006, Helsinki, Nov 2006.

[20] "World health organization: Older adult health and ageing in africa." [Online]. Available: http://www.who.int/healthinfo/survey/ageing/en/index.html

[21] A. Davies, "Ageing and health in the 21st century: an overview," in *Ageing and Health. Proceedings of a WHO Symposium*.

[22] J. Wells, "Protecting and assisting older people in emergencies," *Humanitarian Network Paper: ODI*, 2005.

[23] T. Kosatsky, "The 2003 european heat waves," *EUROPEAN COMMUNICABLE DISEASE JOURNAL*, p. 148, 2005.

[24] "Information society statistical profiles 2009: Africa," International Telecommunication Union, Tech. Rep., 2009.

[25] J. Dai, X. Bai, Z. Yang, Z. Shen, and D. Xuan, "Mobile phone-based pervasive fall detection," *Personal Ubiquitous Comput.*, vol. 14, pp. 633–643, October 2010. [Online]. Available: http://dx.doi.org/10.1007/s00779-010-0292-x

[26] *Egypt State Information Service Year Book*, 2007.

[27] M. Abyad, A. Ashour and M. Abou-Saleh, *In Images in Psychiatry. An Arab Perspective (eds A. Okasha & M. Maj).* World Psychiatric Association, 2001, ch. The scope of psychogeriatrics in the Arab world, pp. 175–188.

[28] "World health organization publications on active ageing." [Online]. Available: http://www.elderlyegypt.com

[29] D. Bertsekas, R. Gallager, P. Humblet, and M. I. of Technology. Center for Advanced Engineering Study, *Data networks.* Prentice-hall New York, 1987.

[30] S. Boyd and L. Vandenberghe, *Convex optimization.* Cambridge Univ Pr, 2004.

[31] Nonin website. [Online]. Available: http://www.nonin.com

[32] A&D Medical website. [Online]. Available: http://www.andonline.com

In: Health Informatics
Editor: Naveen Chilamkurti

ISBN: 978-1-61942-265-0
© 2013 Nova Science Publishers, Inc.

Chapter 2

CONTEXT-AWARE PROCESS AND USER INTERFACE ADAPTATION IN EHEALTH APPLICATIONS — THE LOCA APPROACH

Nadine Fröhlich[1], Andreas Meier[2],
Thorsten Möller[1], Heiko Schuldt[1] and Joël Vogt[2]
[1] Databases and Information Systems Group,
University of Basel, Switzerland
firstname.lastname@unibas.ch
[2] Department of Informatics
University of Fribourg, Switzerland.
firstname.lastname@unifr.ch

ABSTRACT

Mobile devices are becoming more and more popular in a large variety of application domains. In particular, new sensor technologies, powerful mobile devices, and wearable computers in conjunction with wireless communication standards have opened new opportunities in providing customized software solutions. This is particularly relevant in eHealth applications, from pervasive information access in hospital environments to the individual support of patients, both in stationary and home care.

Medical professionals are equipped today with much more powerful hardware and software than some years before. By making use of smart sensors and mobile devices for gathering, processing, and analyzing data, medical doctors and nursing staff are able to get access to relevant information (e.g., patient records) anytime and anywhere in a hospital. Similarly, for patients this technology can be used to provide support which is tailored to their particular needs and impairments.

All these environments are highly dynamic, due to the inherent mobility of users. Therefore, in order to best serve the individual information needs of the different users in eHealth applications, it is of utmost importance to automatically adapt the underlying IT environment to their context – which might change over time when user context evolves. In a digital home environment, this requires the automatic customization of user interfaces and the context-aware adaptation of monitoring workflows for mobile patients. In a hospital environment, such dynamic adaptations will for instance help physicians to automatically retrieve and present the data they need in their current context, without having them to manually search for relevant information (e.g., on a ward round or in an emergency case).

This chapter will give an overview on context-awareness in mobile environments with particular focus on eHealth applications and the special requirements of users in healthcare applications. It will introduce LoCa (a Location and Context-aware eHealth infrastructure), a concrete system that provides a generic software infrastructure, able to dynamically adapt user interfaces and service-based distributed applications (workflows) to the actual context of a user (physician, caregiver, patient, etc.). Furthermore, the chapter will report on the evaluation of the LoCa system based on a prototype system running on smart phones.

Keywords: eHealth, mobile devices, context-awareness, dynamic workflow adaptation, dynamic user interface adaptation.

INTRODUCTION

The last years have seen a vast proliferation of mobile devices, not only for communication purposes, but more and more also for ubiquitous access to information. In particular, such powerful mobile devices with powerful processors and significant local storage capacities, together with new sensor technologies, strongly facilitate the provision of customized software solutions. This is particularly relevant in eHealth applications, from pervasive information access in hospital environments to the individual support of patients, both in stationary and home care. A major requirement in these healthcare applications is that such customization does not need manual intervention, but is rather applied automatically. *Context-aware systems* are the key to providing such customization, especially in cases where users interact with mobile devices. Due to the inherent mobility of users, their context frequently changes, and thus the type of information they need to get access to and the way this information needs to be presented. Based on context information, captured by different kinds of sensors, context-awareness considers the dynamic adaptation of the relevant parts of the software running on a mobile device.

Medical professionals, for instance, are equipped today with much more powerful hardware and software than some years before. By making use of smart sensors and mobile devices for gathering, processing, and analyzing data, medical doctors and nursing staff are able to get access to relevant information, for instance patient records, anytime and anywhere in a hospital. Context-awareness in such applications requires the automatic customization of user interfaces and the automatic adaptation of the workflows which implement the application the user is currently running. In a hospital environment, such dynamic adaptations will for instance help physicians to automatically retrieve and present the data they need in their current context (e.g., on a ward round or in an emergency case) without having to manually search for them, which is a mostly tedious and time-consuming task. Similarly, for patients, this technology can be used to provide support that is tailored to their particular needs and impairments. Especially for patients with cognitive impairments such as dementia patients suffering from Alzheimer's disease, context-aware applications are able to free them from complex interactions with their mobile device while still providing the necessary information they need in their current situation.

This chapter introduces context-awareness and the automatic adaptation of workflow processes and user interfaces on mobile devices. It will also introduce the LoCa system (a Location and Context-aware eHealth infrastructure) which has been implemented to provide a user-friendly and adaptable solution for the automated adaptation of applications in an eHealth environment.

A main feature of LoCa is the consideration of context as a first class citizen. This means that applications and processes as well as user interfaces will be dynamically adapted based on the user's context (e.g., location, activity, schedule, personal preferences, available devices in the user's proximity). LoCa jointly targets applications in home care as well as applications in stationary care. In close collaboration with medical pro-fessionals, different use cases from both areas have been considered and prototypically implemented on top of the LoCa system. From a systems point of view, LoCa makes use of and extends an existing platform for the reliable processing of data streams for health monitoring across fixed and mobile devices [2, 3].

The remainder of this chapter is organized as follows: The next section presents two concrete use cases that show why context-awareness is of very high practical relevance in the eHealth domain. The notion of context and a generic context model are introduced in Section 3. In Section 4, we discuss the dynamic adaptation of workflow processes, and the context-aware adaptation of user interfaces is presented in Section 5. The LoCa system, a prototype implementation that combines the two types of context-aware adaptations presented before, is presented in detail in Section 6. Section 7 concludes.

MOTIVATION

In this section we present two concrete use cases from the healthcare domain: i.) a physician on a ward round in a hospital environment, and ii.) an elderly person with dementia living at home in an ambient assisted living environment. These use cases will provide two sample scenarios that illustrate where and how the techniques that will be presented in the remainder of this chapter can be applied.

A Physician on a Ward Round

On a ward round, the doctor's time should mainly be spent for the interaction with her patients, rather than for searching for relevant data in the clinical information system. Thus, information access in a hospital, in particular retrieving electronic patient records, should be as unobtrusive and efficient as possible.

When a physician enters a sick room and approaches a patient, the physician's mobile phone should automatically display the medical history of the patient (an example is depicted in Figure 1). This first needs proper identification of the patient which can be achieved, for instance, by equipping beds in the sick room with RFID tags or by asking patients to wear a wristband with as RFID tag. This does not only ease the work of the medical experts, it also reduces the chance of making mistakes in identifying patients.

Mobile devices can also support the communication between the physician and the patient. In case the physician wants to share medical images or other multimedia content with her patient for which the mobile device's display is too small, the images should be automatically transferred to the patient's bed-mounted multimedia device or another device with a larger screen nearby. This procedure saves time compared to the conventional procedure, which includes actions such as: login to a stationary computer, open the application, locate the multimedia content to share. What is more, these actions would have to be repeated in more or less the same way in every sick room visited on the ward round. Moreover, the physician should be able to make annotations to the electronic patient records during the ward round. This includes textual information on diagnoses or taking new photos (e.g., of a wound in case of a dermatologist) that are to be linked to individual items of the patient's electronic health record. All annotated information has to be synchronized with the backing clinical information system. The physician might add her annotations instantly during the ward round (thus avoiding additional post-processing back in the office) via different devices such as a smart phone or a tablet PC. Smarts phones are particularly well suited for taking photos for documentation purposes (e.g., on skin irritations), but it is often not comfortable to write text on a smart phone. Tablet PCs, in contrast, are more convenient for text editing but have the disadvantage of a higher weight. Therefore, it would be preferable for the physician to use a tablet PC (or even a stationary computer in the patient's sick room) for writing longer texts. A smart phone that is easy to carry would then mainly be used for identifying the patient, getting most important information about the patient, and for taking short notes. In this case, the physician should be able to seamlessly migrate the state of her application from the smart phone to a stationary device nearby. Ideally, the migration can be done via specific gestures in a fast and user-friendly way.

A Dementia Patient Living at Home

People with dementia are faced with a decline of their cognitive functions, including memory impairment and difficulty to orient in time and space [8]. Assistive applications can support or partly assume impaired cognitive functions by targeting the context dimensions in which the person with dementia experiences difficulties to navigate. Context and context-awareness therefore play a crucial role to tailor applications to individual users' abilities, needs, and current situation. Literature shows that the dementia syndrome itself does not thwart the use of digital assistive applications, at least in the early stages (e.g., [12, 18]). To what extent people with dementia can benefit from assistive applications not only depends on the ability to accommodate the user's cognitive impairments and needs but also on their ability to blend into their personal environment [14, 18]. This limits the scope for standard solutions and demands an understanding of individual users [12, 18].

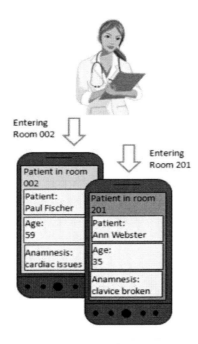

Figure 1. Use Case: Physician on a Ward Round.

Consider the fictive scenario presented in [13] about an elderly couple which is being restricted in their daily activities by dementia. Jon, the husband, who loves being outdoor, was recently diagnosed with dementia. His wife Jane worries for his safety when he is on his own. The traditional tools, a mobile phone and a paper todo list with phone numbers of relatives and close friends, failed to deliver. When Jon is suddenly confused, he forgets to consult the list or to use the phone.

Jane asks their family doctor and friend, Dr. Miller, for help. He suggests to try a mobile assistive application that addresses certain shortcomings of the tools Jon and Jane tried and that is at the same time easy to use. In a first design session, Jon and Jane, Dr. Miller, and a specialized designer discuss several scenarios of use with storyboards. The designer labels context information and system behavior in the storyboard as shown in Figure 2. This information helps to adapt the assistive application to Jon's and Jane's needs.

The resulting application is a context-aware todo list communication application. Jane has to define the place and time of a todo item and add it to Jon's todo list. The system guides Jon to the next item and gives Jane access to Jon's position. Jon can call or send predefined text messages to Jane and other relatives. Additionally, the system informs Jon when he is off route and notifies Jane if he does not react in time to notifications.

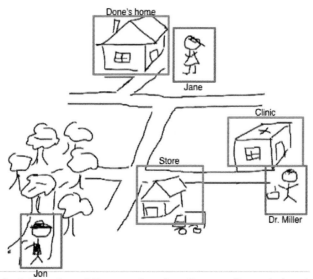

Figure 2. A Storyboard Extract showing Context for assistive Applications in Dementia Care [13].

CONTEXT AND CONTEXT MANAGEMENT

This section will introduce the notion of context and will present a generic model for managing context-related information.

Context and Context-Awareness

With the proliferation of context-aware computing, several definitions of the term context have been introduced and discussed in the literature. The most common definition, which we also adopt in our approach, has been introduced by Day et al. [1]:

> *Context is any information that can be used to characterize the situation of a subject. A subject is a person, place, or object that is considered relevant to the interaction between a user and an application [...] including the user and the application themselves.*

In other words, a situation is generally characterized by all properties of our environment. Context is only a subset; that is, the relevant properties of the complete set of properties. Information can be considered as context in one application while it is not considered being part of the context in another application. That is, nothing is context per se due to its inherent proper– ties [23].

A precise definition of context is especially important for the development of context-aware applications; that is, applications that react on context changes. For this, context has to be continuously sensed and interpreted. This is the basis for the application's adaptation, for instance, adaptation of the dialog information to the current location or to the current user of a device. Ceri [6] describes context-awareness as follows:

> *[...] it can be however interpreted as natural evolution of personalization, addressing not only the user's identity and preferences, but also the usage environment.*

While personalization only handles static context (i.e., context data that infrequently or never change; hence, data that are queried much more frequently than updated), context-awareness in contrast mainly handles dynamic context data. Dynamic context data are frequently updated context data, valid only in a special timeframe, and usually affected by many more updates than queries [11]. Thus, context-awareness extends personalization by taking into account a wider range of properties and it can refer to experience gained in the field of personalization.

Generic Context Model

To enhance an application with the possibility to adapt its behavior based on its context, the proper representation in a convenient and generic context model is needed. Such generic context model has to model important facets of context in a way that offers fast access to and easy understanding of the context data, as well as the possibility to extend and adapt the model to special application domains. Figure 3 depicts a generic model for context data management in entity-relationship notation, with highlighted core entities for better readability, following the well established definition of context by [1] introduced above.

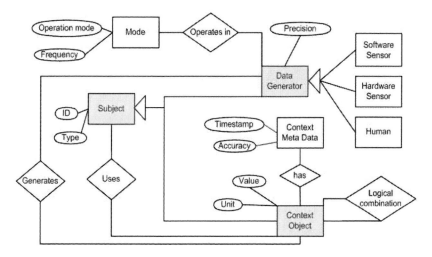

Figure 3. LoCa Context Model.

The entity *Subject* can be a patient, a mobile phone, or an ECG sensor. Conversely, profile data, the medical history, current ECG data, or the current location are examples for context information about a patient. The entity *Context Object* represents the actual context data (e.g., the value of the current location, a document of the medical history, and so on). In order to support data analysis, optional meta data about context objects such as timestamps and data accuracy (which usually depends on the type of sensor used), are captured and stored as well.

The entity *Data Generator* (software sensors, humans, hardware sensors) is designed to capture data about the instrument (sensor) which produces context data: a data generator generates context data about subjects. While many data generators generate atomic data, some sensors may produce compound context objects. For instance, the (GPS) location usually consists of multiple values, such as longitude, latitude, altitude, speed, and bearing. Furthermore, software sensors can combine different kinds of context objects to compose higher level context data. An alarm in case of cardiac problems could be combined of information about the current activity of a patient and his current ECG values. This is covered in the model by means of the relationship *logical combination*.

The context model is able to handle different kinds of context objects, including nested context objects. An important feature of the context model is its rather simple, yet expressive structure. It is powerful enough to cover different context objects, but it can also be extended by adding new data generators and thus also new context objects, if necessary.

CONTEXT-AWARE PROCESS ADAPTATION

This section starts with a brief introduction to workflows and workflow management and points out problems that arise when traditional static workflows are used in a dynamic environment in which a user's context is subject to frequent changes. Since dynamic workflows can solve most of the problems occurring in these environments, different approaches to dynamically adapt processes and workflows are presented. Dynamic workflows that use context information for adaptation are called *context-aware workflows*. This section concludes with a description of context-aware workflows and their implementation.

Static Workflows

Workflows represent real-world processes (e.g., a ward round in a hospital) by defining activities and their order of execution within these processes (also known as control flow) and by defining the information exchange between these activities (also known as data flow). In an eHealth context, the use of workflows offers several advantages over ad hoc applications, in particular in terms of the documentation and standardization of processes, and their automation.

The traditional approach to workflow management considers static workflows whose activities, control flow and data flow is known in advance, prior to their invocation. This is particularly beneficial for routine tasks with high repetition rates such as bank transfers. Nevertheless, such static workflows come to their limitations when applications are to be modeled and executed by means of processes i.) have a complex structure, ii.) change often because of enhancements in processes, exceptions, or unforeseen events, or iii.) their structure cannot be known before run-time. Note that the third case can be seen as special case of the second case.

Workflow management usually follows a two phase approach. In the first phase (build-time), a workflow is defined. This includes the set of constituent activities, their order of execution, and the exchange of data between activities. In the second phase, the workflow description is used as a blueprint for enacting several independent workflow instances of the same type at run-time. Usually, modifications of workflows are only allowed at build-time, and then only if there are no running instances. Hence, when working with static workflows, people will try to avoid changes and will rather attempt to model every detail and every eventuality within the workflow description. This renders workflows complex and significantly increases modeling efforts. However, assumptions made at build-time might become obsolete at run-time. Therefore, the control and data flow of a workflow either have to be completely known a priory, or cannot be modeled at all, if they are not static.

For healthcare applications (see for instance Section 2), traditional, static approaches to workflow management are far too rigid. The reason is that such applications can be characterized by a potentially large number of i.) different ways to achieve a goal which results in complex structures when modeled by means of static workflows (e.g., different devices can be used to meter blood pressure or to show patient records); ii.) dynamic and continuous changes (e.g., new devices, or treatment methods); iii.) exceptions or unforeseen events (e.g., abnormal deviations in sensed physiological data that may require alternative medication); and iv.) decisions that can be made only at run-time (e.g., results of tests cause different subsequent tests or treatments).

Dynamic and Context-Aware Workflows

Dynamic workflows aim at offering a higher degree of flexibility by allowing for structural changes not only at build-time but also at run-time – in the latter case, this usually requires that no running workflow instances exist. As a side effect of this added flexibility by run-time changes, workflow descriptions are usually less complex as not all choices have to be explicitly modeled inside the workflow.

Some approaches to dynamic workflow management can additionally handle changes of workflow definitions of instantiated (i.e., currently running) workflows. This is done by means of migration (i.e., a running instance will be migrated in order to follow the new description for the remainder of its execution). Migration covers evolutionary changes and can be done by i.) aborting all affected instances, ii.) aborting all affected instances with subsequent automatic restart, iii.) continuing to execute existing instances that follow the previous definition and launching new instances according the updated definition, and iv.) transferring running instances to the new defini‐ tion [20].

When a necessary change does not affect future instances, run-time changes of individual instances should be preferred over build-time changes. According to [22] there are two kinds of run-time changes dynamic workflows can offer: process adaptation and built-in flexibility.

Process adaptation is based on modification operations like add, delete, or swap of workflow fragments. Workflow fragments are connected subsets of activities, together with control and data flow dependencies. This is a very flexible approach that needs little assumptions and no pre-planning for the implementation of modification operations. Nevertheless, it is a profound change of the workflow instance and the correctness of the instance needs to be verified to make sure that it can be properly executed.

Built-in flexibility supports the exchange of fragments within a workflow. Types of built-in flexibility are late binding, late modeling, and late composition [22]. For late binding and late modeling, a workflow consisting of both placeholder activities and concrete activities is defined at build-time. At run-time, placeholder activities are replaced by concrete fragments (activities and associated control flow specifications). While for late binding concrete fragments that will dynamically be added can already be defined at build-time, late modeling assumes that the concrete fragments to be inserted into a workflow description are also modeled at run-time. In both cases, it has to be specified a priori which activities are placeholder activities (and are therefore flexible as they can be replaced at run-time) and thus where dynamic behavior can be added to a workflow. Besides these two approaches that require pre-planning but no or little verification effort at run-time, there is a yet another approach to built-in flexibility, called late composition. The approach needs verification at run-time. It is characteristic for offering the highest degree of decision deferral: At build-time, process fragments are specified; at run-time, the process instance is composed of these fragments. Thus, all the work for composing the workflow is shifted from build-time to run-time.

In summary, the later the decision making takes place, the more flexible a workflow is – but the more work has to be done at run-time. There are different kinds of dynamic workflows but all of them have in common that they have to provide the following features [15]:

1) the identification of relevant changes in the current situation, based on the sensed context,
2) the dynamic adaptation of workflows according to context changes, and
3) the verification of the adaptation, to make sure that the workflow execution can be seamlessly continued, without run-time failures.

When striving for automated execution of dynamic workflows, the workflows' context should be used for decision making. Such context-aware workflows have to solve the same problems as dynamic workflows but in an automated way based on context information used for triggering dynamic adaptation.

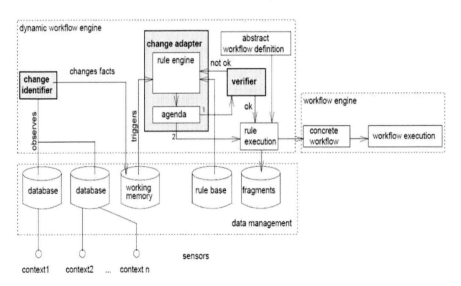

Figure 4. Context-aware Workflow System.

Implementation of Context-Aware Workflows

The features provided in the previous section guide the implementation of a system able to dynamically and automatically adapt workflows to evolving user context (see Figure 4).

Identification of Context Changes: to recognize a context change, context has to be acquired. To find out whether new context implies the adaptation of a running workflow instance, the new context has to be compared to the most recent context metering. Therefore, for building a context-aware workflow system, hardware and software sensors for acquiring relevant context are needed as well as a data store for storing these data (see Section 3.2). Furthermore, a dynamic workflow system needs a component able to identify and compare subsequent context information.

Dynamic Adaptation to Context Changes: context changes can lead to another execution path of the workflow; that is, to an adaptation of the workflow. After a change has been identified, components for triggering and executing the adaptations are needed. A way to automatically adapt the workflow to the new execution path is the usage of rule engines for identifying, based on predefined rules, the necessary changes. Rule engines are well suited for these applications since they are designed to allow for efficient inference in complex systems consisting of a large number of rules. This means that the large number of alternative executions which have to be explicitly modeled in static workflows is represented as a large set of adaptation rules (together with conditions when these changes are applicable) in the case of dynamic workflows.

Verification of the Adaptation: it is necessary to guarantee that the remainder of a workflow instance, after adaptation, can be correctly executed. This requires a dedicated component for verification which has to verify a workflow instance right after adaptation, prior to the continuation of execution.

Discussion

Context-aware workflow systems extend dynamic workflow systems by incorporating sensors for capturing context data, databases for persistently storing context data, and components that identify context changes. In addition, software components such as rule engines are required for adapting workflows by relating pre-defined workflow fragments and context changes (events) under certain conditions. Finally, functionality for the verification of adapted workflows needs to be provided. A generic system architecture for context-aware workflow systems is depicted in Figure 4.

In practice, sensed data is not always in a form directly usable for dynamic adaptation. For instance, if several distributed context databases are used, context data first need to be integrated and possibly also cleansed or generalized. As an example, consider modern thermometers that can also meter barometric pressure, even though not all applications will need this additional sensor data. Different position measuring instruments do not have the same precision – to find the actual position of a user, data from different sensors might have to be combined and thus context data first need to be integrated (after transformation). Finally, it can be necessary to generalize context data (e.g., to characterize metered temperature data as warm, cold, and so on). Therefore, according to the context model presented in Section 3.2, additional meta data accuracy and support logical combination is stored together with raw context data.

While current approaches to context-aware workflow management rely on sensed context data for adaptation, it might be interesting to predict upcoming context changes based on past changes, and to anticipate adaptations of workflows. This requires the continuous analysis of stored context data and thus the monitoring of their evolution over time [21].

CONTEXT-AWARE USER INTERFACE ADAPTATION

The rising computer literacy rate among the general population and the realization of ubiquitous computing extends the reach of digital medical systems beyond the physical realm of medical organizations. This encourages a shift from seeing the medical professionals as the sole users of digital medical devices to include patients as well [19].

Providing user interfaces that are sensitive to their users' situation and behave accordingly is important for both medical professionals and patients. Context-awareness in the adaptation of user interfaces has the potential to develop and run applications that are able to better adjust to users' preferences and changing needs.

In general, Calvary et al. [5] identify different dimensions in the interaction between human users and systems: *user*, *device*, and *environment*. The user model contains user attributes that influence the system. Adaptation to the user's needs (static context) considers individual traits of the user such as age, current location, and emotions [4]. Adapting the device in contrast would consider the physical device and software platform the framework is running on. Attributes include the CPU speed, the screen size, or the operating system [17]. The environment model contains information about surroundings in which the application runs such as illumination or noise (dynamic context) [5].

Adapting User Interfaces to their User's Context

The adaption of user interfaces to the context of use can occur at different stages [5]. Static adaption occurs at build-time, hence before the system is executed. An example is the configuration for multiple types of display sizes or specification of user preferences and abilities, such as language, color, or font size.

Dynamic adaption on the other hand occurs for adaptations that cannot be known beforehand. The system providing dynamic adaptations is aware of the environment it operates in and reacts to changes in the context. The system can present context to the user, either to negotiate further steps or to provide the user with situation-dependent information. Alternatively, the system can react to the current context without consulting the user first by automatically executing functions [7].

A hybrid approach combines both forms, therefore including known contextual information before the system runs and specifying the system's reactions to changes in the current context.

Abstraction Layers of User Interfaces

Context can influence various aspects of user interfaces. The Cameleon reference framework proposes four abstraction layers at which context can manifest itself in user interfaces [5]. At the most abstract level, the task model defines the functional aspects and objects of a user interface. An often referred task model is the ConcurTaskTrees (CTT) [16]. CTT has four types of tasks: i.) system tasks that are conducted by the system alone, ii.) user tasks that are only performed by a user, iii.) interaction tasks in which the user and the system collaborate, and iv.) abstract tasks that contain children of the former task types. A CTT task has several properties including the name of the task, whether it is used to edit or view data, input and output objects, data objects and actions that can be attached to the task, an iteration attribute as well as pre- and post-conditions. At the same level in the Cameleon reference framework, the concepts model describes the information objects that are manipulated by the tasks.

The abstract user interface provides a canonical description of the user interface of the tasks and the domain objects, independent of an interaction modality. The concrete user interface describes the abstract user interface for a specific type of presentation, independent of any implementation. The final user interface is an actual presentation of the concrete user interface to the user, for example, as an HTML page.

A CONCRETE EXAMPLE: THE LOCA SYSTEM

This section introduces and discusses in detail the LoCa system that seamlessly combines process and user interface adaptation together with local context management on mobile devices [9]. LoCa has been developed at the Universities of Basel and Fribourg in close collaboration with medical experts and has been funded by the Hasler foundation.[1]

Architecture of the LoCa System

Context-aware application behavior requires that information gathered from distributed sensors (data generators) is stored in a global, distributed database that instantiates the context model presented in Section 3.2. Prior to inserting raw sensor data into this database, data need to be cleansed and transformed into the global schema. Since context data are a vital input for all LoCa applications, the context data management layer forms the basis of the LoCa system architecture depicted in Figure 5.

On top of context management, all LoCa applications are defined by means of workflow processes. The basic assumption is that functionality is available in the form of (Web) services so that workflows can be defined by combining existing services. Since complete workflows again have a service interface, service composition can be applied recursively. A crucial part of this layer is dynamic workflow adaptation. This layer makes use of the raw sensor data and their relationships stored in the context layer. The top-most layer of

---

[1] http://www.haslerstiftung.ch/en/home

the LoCa architecture deals with the dynamic generation and adaptation of user interfaces. Again, this layer directly accesses the underlying context data management.

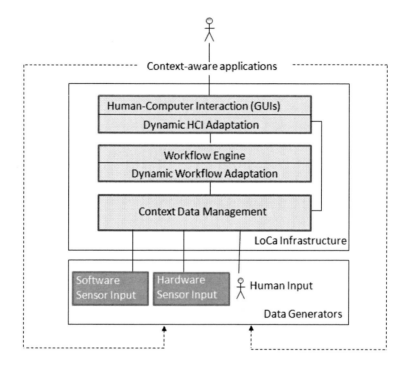

Figure 5. LoCa System Architecture.

The LoCa architecture offers a unified interface for (individual, user-defined or pre-existing) workflow-based applications. According to the context model, LoCa workflow-based applications themselves can be considered software sensors (i.e., they might produce context objects that are subsequently needed for dynamic adaptation).

Implementation of the LoCa System

To identify tools suited for efficient implementation of the LoCa architecture introduced in Section 6.1, different data management systems have been analyzed in a benchmark and different rule engines have been evaluated.

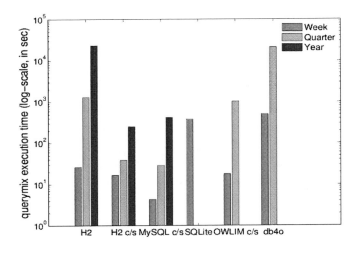

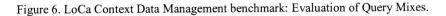

Figure 6. LoCa Context Data Management benchmark: Evaluation of Query Mixes.

LoCa Context Data Management Layer

For context-aware eHealth applications, fast access to context data is required in order to apply dynamic adaptations on-line, without relying on network connections to a remote server. This means that all relevant context data (raw and derived data) needs to be stored locally on the user's mobile device.

In order to evaluate the efficiency of different data stores on mobile devices for use by the LoCa system, a *benchmark for mobile context-aware applications* has been designed and implemented [10]. The benchmark set-up is driven by an eHealth use case and considers context queries, as they are needed for finding out relevant context changes, as well as updates of the user's current context. In the evaluation, the performance of relational databases and object-oriented databases running on the Android Nexus One smart phone has been analyzed. In addition, for comparison, also RDF triple stores in client/server mode have been considered. To evaluate the local storage capabilities of mobile devices, different context data sets have been considered. For the latter, the benchmarks simulate the use of mobile devices in context-aware applications for the period of a week, a month, and a year. These settings essentially differ in the volume of raw context data that are accumulated over the periods considered.

The actual benchmark considers context queries and concurrent updates to the context data store as users are considered to be mobile (i.e., their context may change) while the system is applying dynamic adaptations at the same time. The benchmark results consider the performance of selected queries and the average performance of all queries in the query mix (see Figure 6).

From the systems that have been evaluated, relational data stores in client/server mode performed best, especially for large data sets. However, for the smaller data sets, embedded relational databases have shown reasonable performance in order to be used for on-line adaptations. As in most context-aware applications only the most recent context is relevant and changes only need to be compared to recent context, it is fair to assume that context stores can be pruned. Thus the volume of data to be maintained on the mobile device is limited. More details on the benchmark set-up and the evaluation results can be found in [10].

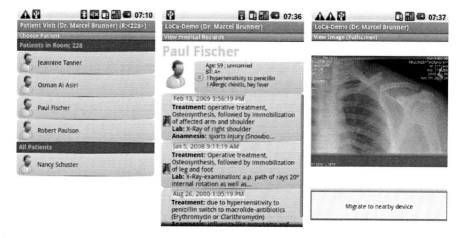

(a) Patients in sick room 228   (b) Patient record   (c) X-ray in patient record

Figure 7. Screenshots of the LoCa Demonstrator.

Tool Support for Dynamic Adaptations

The LoCa system focuses on run-time changes and adaptations without manual intervention. To his end, rules for automated adaptation, in particular for workflows, are provided. That is, automated fragment selection or evaluated on the mobile device.

A detailed analysis of existing rule engines, including the development of a prototype application from an eHealth environment (ward round use case, see Section 2.1), has shown that compatibility with mobile devices is still limited. In order to meet the performance requirements of LoCa, a remote full-fledged rule engine is still to be preferred over a rule engine running on a mobile device as the latter is constrained by limited local resources.

LoCa Prototype System

To better support the discussion on the LoCa concepts with healthcare professionals, the LoCa project started with early prototype development in order to demonstrate and show the main project ideas and also to refine the use cases that have been implemented. This prototype (and also the benchmark and performance evaluations presented in Section 6.2) are based on two generations of Android smart phones: first, a T-Mobile G1 (HTC Dream) running Google Android version 1.6, equipped with a Qualcomm MSM7201A processor with 528 MHz and 192 MB RAM and second, a Nexus One (N1) phone running Android version 2.1. The latter comes with 512MB RAM, and a Qualcomm QSD8250 CPU with 1 GHz.

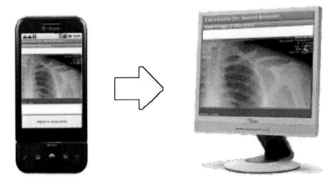

Figure 8. Application Migration in LoCa: Switching X-Rays from a Mobile Phone to a Stationary Computer.

From a functional point of view, the LoCa demonstrator follows the ward round application presented in Section 2.1. Figure 7 (a) shows the mobile phone's screen that a physician sees when she enters a patient room. On this screen, the physician can select the patient she wants to examine (if there are many). After selection, an overview on the patient record (retrieved from the hospital's clinical information system) is displayed (Figure 7(b)). The patient record entries are ordered by date. By selecting a treatment, a detailed view on this treatment process is shown, and the physician is able to add and annotate information on her device which is then propagated back to the underlying clinical IS.

Usually, multimedia documents such as ECG plots, X-rays, or videos are attached to a patient record. These documents can be presented in the first place on a smart phone. However, especially when it comes to the identification of details within these documents, the visualization on larger screens will be preferred. For this reason, LoCa offers the seamless migration of application state from one device to another as part of the dynamic, context-aware adaptation (see Figure 8). Therefore, detected devices in the user's proximity that can serve as target for application migration are part of the current context.

Besides the migration of multimedia documents, a migration of application states can be meaningful, especially for the physician to take diagnoses notes with comfortable input devices and large screens. To support such migrations, an application-independent library able to enhance any (smart phone) application by migration functionality has been developed. In order not to disturb the user's interaction with the system due to unintentional, automated migration, the actual migration process is initiated by dedicated gestures.

CONCLUSION

This chapter has presented a concrete approach to providing context-aware applications for information access on mobile devices in an eHealth environment. The inherent mobility of users implies that their context is subject to frequent changes, and thus also their specific needs in terms of access to and presentation of information. Context-awareness aims at automatically adapting the key software components relevant for information access and presentation: workflow processes which encapsulate the application logic, and user interfaces.

Context-aware adaptations have been designed, implemented, and evaluated in cooperation with medical professionals in the LoCa project. From an end user's point of view, context-aware applications are highly appreciated as they free users from dealing with tedious systems tasks (customization, re-configuration) and most importantly allow them to focus exclusively on their professional activities. From a developer's point of view, complexity is shifted from the implementation of system components (UI programming or workflow specification) to the identification and definition of modular elements and the specification of rules indicating how they can be applied (workflow fragments, rules, story boards).

It is expected that context-aware applications are becoming more and more popular, especially when context-awareness is supported by sophisticated software systems, even more powerful mobile devices, and a larger variety of dynamic adaptations (e.g., the delegation of tasks between users, support for collaborative applications, automated and case-specific data sharing).

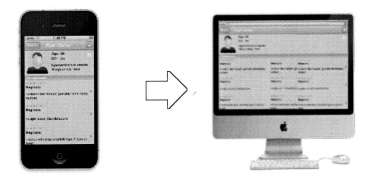

Figure 9. LoCa Demonstrator: Migration of Application States.

ACKNOWLEDGMENTS

This work has been funded by the Hasler Foundation. The authors like to thank the healthcare experts who contributed to the requirements analysis for the LoCa system: H. Mengisen, L. Wagner, J. Moerlen (Merian Iselin Hospital Basel), S. Reichlin (Siemens), A. Dyson, H. Kollmar (MedGate), H. Behrendt, U. Genewein, F. Thieringer, D. Pulvermüller (University Hospital Basel).

REFERENCES

[1]   G. Abowd, A. Dey, P. Brown, et al. Towards a Better Understanding of Context and Context-Awareness. In: *Proceedings of the International Symposium on Handheld and Ubiquitous Computing*, pages 304–307, London, UK, 1999. Springer.

[2]   G. Brettlecker and H. Schuldt. The OSIRIS-SE (Stream-Enabled) Infrastructure for Reliable Data Stream Management on Mobile Devices. In: *Proceedings of the ACM SIGMOD International Conference on Management of Data (SIGMOD 2007)*, pages 1097–1099, Beijing, China, June 2007. ACM.

[3]   G. Brettlecker and H. Schuldt. Reliable Distributed Data Stream Management in Mobile Environments. *Information Systems*, 36(3):618–643, 2011.

[4]   P. Brusilovsky and E. Millán. User Models for Adaptive Hypermedia and Adaptive Educational Systems. In P. Brusilovsky, A. Kobsa, and W. Nejdl, editors, *The Adaptive Web*, volume 4321 of Lecture Notes in Computer Science, pages 3–53. Springer, 2007.

[5]   G. Calvary, J. Coutaz, D. Thevenin, Q. Limbourg, L. Bouillon, and J. Vanderdonckt. A Unifying Reference Framework for Multi-Target User Interfaces. *Interacting with Computers*, 15(3):289–308, 2003.

[6]   S. Ceri, F. Daniel, M. Matera, Federico, and M. Facca. Model-driven Development of Context-aware Web Applications. *ACM Transactions on Internet Technology (TOIT)*, 7:2, 2007.

[7]   A. K. Dey and G. D. Abowd. Towards a Better Understanding of Context and Context-Awareness. In: *CHI 2000 Workshop on the What, Who, Where, When, and How of Context-Awareness*, volume 4, pages 1–6, 2000.

[8]   B. Draper. Dealing with Dementia: a Guide to Alzheimer's Disease and other Dementias. Allen & Unwin, Crows Nest, N.S.W., 2004.

[9]   N. Fröhlich, A. Meier, T. Möller, M. Savini, H. Schuldt, and J. Vogt. LoCa Towards a Context-aware Infrastructure for eHealth Applications. In: *Proceedings of the 15th International Conference on Distributed Multimedia Systems (DMS'09)*, Redwood City, CA, USA, Sept. 2009.

[10] N. Fröhlich, S. Rose, T. Möller, and H. Schuldt. A benchmark for context data management in mobile context-aware applications. In: *Proceedings of the 4th International Workshop on Personalized Access, Profile Management, and Context Awareness in Databases (PersDB'2010)*, Singapore, 9 2010.

[11] M. Grossmann, M. Bauer, N. Honle, U.-P. Kappeler, D. Nicklas, and T. Schwarz. Efficiently Managing Context Information for Large-Scale Scenarios. In: *Proceedings of the 3rd IEEE International Conference on Pervasive Computing and Communications (PERCOM'05)*, pages 331–340, Washington, DC, USA, 2005. IEEE Computer Society.

[12] S. Lauriks, A. Reinersmann, H. G. Van der Roest, F. Meiland, R. J. Davies, F. Moelaert, M. D. Mulvenna, C. D. Nugent, and R. M. Dröes. Review of ICT-based Services for identified unmet Needs in People with Dementia. *Ageing Research Reviews*, 6(3):223–246, 2007.

[13] N. Mahmud, J. Vogt, K. Luyten, K. Slegers, J. Van Den Bergh, and K. Coninx. Dazed and Confused Considered Normal: an Approach to Create Interactive Systems for People with Dementia. In: *Proceedings of the 3rd International Conference on Human-Centred Software Engineering (HCSE'10)*, volume 6409 of Lecture Notes in Computer Science, pages 119–134, Reykjavik, Iceland, 2010. Springer-Verlag.

[14] A. F. Monk. Simple, Social, Ethical and Beautiful: Requirements for UIs in the Home. In: *Proceedings of the 9th Australasian User Interface Conference (AUIC'08)*, pages 3–9, Darlinghurst, Australia, 2008. Australian Computer Society, Inc.

[15] R. Müller, U. Greiner, and E. Rahm. A$_{GENT}$W$_{ORK}$: a Workflow System supporting rule-based Workflow Adaptation. *Data & Knowledge Engineering*, 51(2):223–256, 2004.

[16] F. Paterno, C. Mancini, and S. Meniconi. ConcurTaskTrees: A Diagrammatic Notation for Specifying Task Models. In: *Human-Computer Interaction: Interact'97*, page 362. Chapman & Hall, 1997.

[17] J. Rabin, A. Trasatti, and R. Hanrahan. Device Description Repository Core Vocabulary 1k, 2008. http://www.w3.org/2005/MWI/DDWG/ Drafts/ corevocabulary/latest.

[18] L. Robinson, K. Brittain, S. Lindsay, D. Jackson, and P. Olivier. Keeping in touch everyday (kite) project: developing assistive technologies with people with dementia and their carers to promote independence. *International Psychogeriatrics*, 21(03):494–502, 2008.

[19] M. Savini, H. Stormer, and A. Meier. Integrating Context Information in a Mobile Environment using the eSana Framework. In: *Proceedings of the 2nd European Conference on eHealth (ECEH)*, Oldenburg, Germany, Oct. 2007.

[20] M. Schonenberg, R. Mans, N. Russell, and W. van der Aalst. Towards a Taxonomy of Process Flexibility (Extended Version). *BPM Center Report BPM-07-11*, BPM-07-11, 2007.

[21] S. Sigg, S. Haseloff, and K. David. Prediction of Context Time Series. In: *Proceedings of the 5th Workshop on Applications of Wireless Communications (WAWC'07)*, Lappeenranta, Finnland, 2007.

[22] B. Weber, S. Rinderle, and M. Reichert. Change Patterns and Change Support Features in Process-Aware Information Systems. In: *Proceedings of the 19th Conference on Advanced Information Systems Engineering (CAiSE 2007)*, pages 574–588. Springer LNCS, Trondheim, Norway, June 2007.

[23] T. Winograd. Architectures for Context. *Human-Computer Interaction*, 16(2-4):401–419, 2001.

In: Health Informatics
Editor: Naveen Chilamkurti

ISBN: 978-1-61942-265-0
© 2013 Nova Science Publishers, Inc.

Chapter 3

ENHANCING NETWORK PATIENT CAPACITY IN A WLAN FOR HEALTHCARE MONITORING

*Di Lin and Fabrice Labeau**
Department of Electrical and Computer Engineering,
McGill University, Canada

Abstract

From the perspective of network design, network patient capacity, which we define as the number of patients that one wireless local area network deployment can support, is a critical design criterion and performance metric for wireless healthcare systems. In this chapter, we first introduce the background of wireless healthcare systems, including the motivations, the categories, the architectures, and the challenges of wireless healthcare in-hospital monitoring systems. Building on the specific characteristics of the wireless healthcare monitoring environment, we study network patient capacity in view of two particular issues for wireless systems, namely, imperfect channel state information (CSI) and electromagnetic interference (EMI).

PACS 05.45-a, 52.35.Mw, 96.50.Fm

*E-mail address: di.lin2@mail.mcgill.ca, fabrice.labeau@mcgill.ca

Keywords: resource allocation, wireless healthcare monitoring

AMS Subject Classification: 53D, 37C, 65P

1. Background

The world health report shows that the proportion of investment in healthcare to Gross Domestic Product (GDP) has annually increased by 0.1% in a wide range of the member countries of World Health Organization (WHO) [1]. The governments expect to improve the quality of healthcare by increasing financial support. Moreover, the rapid development of wireless communication and computing technologies has provided a potential way of improving the quality of healthcare. Therefore, the healthcare monitoring with the aid of wireless communication and computing technologies shows great promise.

Rashvand et al. in [2] clarify three concepts with respect to wireless healthcare monitoring, including telemedicine (TLM), telehealth (TLH) and E-health. TLM may be as simple as two clinicians discussing a case over the telephone [3], or as complex as using satellite networks to conduct a real-time consultation between health professionals in two different countries [4]. Generally, TLM is defined as the provision of healthcare information with the aid of advanced telecommunication and computing technologies [4]. It mainly serves patient healthcare by transferring medical information through internet or telecommunication networks. While TLM focuses on the healthcare for patients, TLH has a broader definition. Besides the aspect of patient healthcare, TLH encompasses healthcare education, public health as well as the development of health systems [2]. In comparison with TLM and TLH, E-health has an even broader definition. It encompasses a range of services that are at the edge of medicine and information technology. Specifically, E-health includes informational, educational, and commercial aspects of health services [5].

In this chapter, we only focus on healthcare monitoring systems (HMS), which are a part of TLM related to clinical medicine. Besides clinical medicine, other applications of TLM include prevention, remote diagnosis, remote treatment, disease management, etc. [6]. The relationship of HMS, TLM, TLH and E-health is shown in Fig.1.

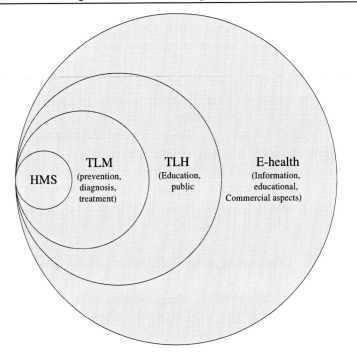

Figure 1. Relationship of healthcare monitoring systems (HMS), telemedicine (TLM), telehealth (TLH), and E-health.

1.1. Motivations of healthcare monitoring systems

As a rapid developing application of clinical medicine, healthcare monitoring is mainly motivated by the issues of population aging, medical errors, inconsistent treatment, and treatment delay. Specifically, the rise of aging population, which is the main crowd in need of healthcare, is widespread across the world. The number of individuals over 65 is forecasted to be approximately 761 million worldwide by 2025 [1]. Population aging burdens the healthcare system because of the scarcity of healthcare staff. Secondly, medical errors in current healthcare monitoring systems would result in numerous unnecessary deaths. A medical error occurs when a health provider chooses an inappropriate method of care or executes a right solution of care incorrectly. In the hospital settings of U.S., medical errors are estimated to cause 44, 000 to 200, 000 unnecessary deaths and $1,000,000$ excess injuries each year [7]. Additionally, people nowadays are always on business trips around the world. They cannot receive continuous medical treatment due to the inconsistent quality of healthcare in different places [2]. The treatment records of a particular patient at a hospital cannot be accessed by doctors at another hospital, so the patient may receive inefficient treatment due to a lack of previous treatment records. Finally, patients, especially those living in isolated communities and remote regions, have to wait several days or even months to see a clinician or specialist who can provide an accurate and complete examination. This delay sometimes causes the death of patients [2]. Moreover, when clinicians or specialists provide professional treatment, they have to do other things at the same time, such as organizing and managing the medical records. In short, they are distracted from their most important work [8].

To improve the quality of healthcare monitoring, researchers and technical staff attempt to apply wireless communication and computing technologies for healthcare monitoring systems. These wireless healthcare monitoring systems may improve the healthcare quality and avoid unnecessary deaths by collecting patients' information, detecting abnormal cases, and alerting the healthcare staff once abnormal cases occur.

1.2.   Categories and architecture of healthcare monitoring systems

Healthcare monitoring systems have rapidly advanced in past decades due to the four motivators in Section 1.1. Building on their coverage, healthcare monitoring systems can mainly be classified into two categories: in-hospital monitoring systems [9, 10] and remote monitoring systems [11, 12]. In-hospital monitoring systems serve inpatients who usually require intensive care. Once an abnormal case occurs, the healthcare staff must be alerted in time since a delay of even a few seconds may sometimes mean a loss of life. Remote monitoring systems mainly serve the elderly or chronic patients, and emergent cases seldom occur.

In an in-hospital monitoring system or a remote monitoring system, the network traffic is similar, generally being composed of nonrealtime and real-time traffic [13]. Vergados et al. present [13] that the nonrealtime traffic mainly includes querying medical papers and files as well as transferring medical routine data, while real-time traffic covers the audio and video applications as well as various messages.

In an in-hospital monitoring system, the medical data, such as electrocardio-gram (ECG), breathing, body temperature, blood pressure, oxygen saturation, etc., are usually packetized before transmission. Cypher et al. in [14] take pack-etizing ECG as an example to illustrate the process of data packetization, shown in Fig.2. After packetization, medical data would be transmitted in the network, and the requirements of transmitting particular biosignals are shown in Table.1.

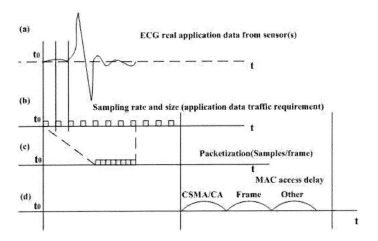

Figure 2. Packetization process of medical data [14] (©2006 IEEE, reproduced with permission).

From the perspectives of bandwidth requirement, network coverage, and network architecture, Cypher et al. select body area network (BAN), wireless local are network (WLAN), and wide area network (WAN) as the most appro-priate networks for healthcare monitoring [14]. Specifically, a BAN [15] is employed to transmit medical data from sensors to patient computing devices, a WLAN is employed to transmit data from patient computing devices to the server, and a WAN is employed to transmit data from the residences of patients to hospitals. The architecture of healthcare monitoring systems is shown in Fig.3, and the range marked by dashed lines represents the wireless network employed in in-hospital monitoring systems, on which this chapter focuses.

Table 1. Typical requirements for biosignal transmission [13] (©2006 IEEE, reproduced with permission).

Biomedical Measurements	Voltage range (V)	Number of sensors	Bandwidth (Hz)	Sample rate (samples/s)	Information rate (bytes/s)
ECG	$0.4 - 5m$	$5 - 9$	$0.01 - 250$	1250	12
Heart sound	Extremely small	$2 - 4$	$5 - 2000$	10000	12
Heart rate	$0.5 - 4m$	2	$0.4 - 5$	25	24
EEG	$2 - 200\mu$	20	$0.5 - 70$	350	12
EMG	$0.1 - 5m$	2+	$0 - 10000$	50000	12
Respiratory rate	Small	1	$0.1 - 10$	50	16
Temperature of body	$0.1m$	1+	$0 - 1$	5	16

1.3. Challenges in the network for healthcare

As mentioned in section 1.1, healthcare monitoring systems can be classified into in-hospital monitoring systems and remote monitoring systems. Before full-scale implementation of these systems, there are a number of challenges that have to be addressed. These challenges mainly include device training concerns, management issues, and demanding technologies for wireless healthcare [17].

Over the past decades, healthcare has focused on standards of care building on studies in epidemiology. A clinician would follow a standard diagnostic and treatment process and keep a standard record for a certain type of patients. However, large cohort studies do not take into account the difference of individuals within a population. Personalized medicine is proposed to seek for an objective basis taking into account individual difference. In personalized medicine, individual difference is an important consideration of diagnosis and treatment for a particular patient. In a wireless healthcare monitoring system, a device would automatically make the diagnosis and treatment plan for a patient. How to train the device to fulfill the requirements of personalized medicine would be a great challenge.

Additionally, for wireless healthcare monitoring to be successful, piles of management issues need to be solved, including better protection of patients' privacy when they using wireless monitoring technologies, training the healthcare staff to become proficient in operating wireless monitoring devices, and resolving the legal and regulatory issues with respect to wireless healthcare,

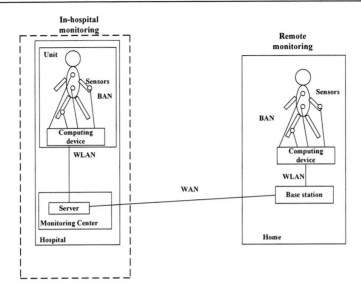

Figure 3. Architecture of healthcare monitoring systems [16] (©2010 IEEE, reproduced with permission).

etc. [17].

Finally, to meet the technical challenges of wireless healthcare monitoring, some advanced telecommunications and information technologies need to be reshaped. Specifically, technical challenges include concerns of designing devices and issues of data transmission in the network. The devices in a wireless healthcare system include sensing devices, tracking devices, and computing devices. Sensing devices need to be small, light and portable. They should have little impact on the daily life of patients, and be reliable for a long time under various conditions [6]. Tracking devices are especially beneficial to monitoring the patients with any psychological disorder. They need continuous attention and slight carelessness in their caring may lead to any misfortune. For healthcare monitoring, a tracking device should be real-time and with high tracking accuracy to enable healthcare staff to continuously follow the patients' positions. However, the design of a tracking device real-time and with high tracking accuracy is a serious challenge. To help clinicians monitor patients efficiently, computing devices in a wireless healthcare system must face the challenges of collecting and storing a significant amount of medical data, detecting abnormal conditions of patients, and alerting the healthcare staff for medical intervention.

Wireless networks applied for healthcare monitoring may include WPAN, WLAN, WAN, Satellite networks, and so on. Reliability and transmission delay in these networks should be of primary importance, while other considerations, such as network throughput, may become secondary [11]. In a wireless healthcare system, several issues may have influence on reliability and transmission delay, mainly including the handover of data between heterogeneous networks, the interference of WLAN and BAN at the frequencies around 2.4 GHz, and the limited resources to satisfy the demands of monitoring quite a few patients in clinics or hospitals.

In this chapter, we center on the last issue. As the solution to the problem of monitoring numerous patients subject to limited resources, we will present the schemes of resource allocation in the following sections.

1.4. Introduction to wireless local area networks

The design of WLAN for healthcare monitoring is based on a set of standards: 802.11. In the past decades, IEEE 802.11 group has released a series of standards, mainly including IEEE 802.11-1997, IEEE 802.11a, IEEE 802.11b, IEEE 802.11g, and IEEE 802.11n. Their frequency bands, data rate, modulation schemes, and coverage are illustrated in Table.2. Among these 802.11 standards, the most widely used are IEEE 802.11b and IEEE 802.11g. Both of IEEE 802.11b and IEEE 802.11g operate at 2.4 GHz instead of 5 GHz, at which IEEE 802.11a operate. Due to a larger wavelength of 802.11b and 802.11g signals, they could lower absorption when penetrating walls [18]. Thus, IEEE 802.11b and IEEE 802.11g can operate in a wider range than IEEE 802.11a.

IEEE 802.11n evolves from IEEE 802.11b and IEEE 802.11g, and it is designed to raise data rate [19]. In IEEE 802.11n, two advanced technologies are employed: one is multiple-input multiple-output (MIMO) technology in the physical layer, and the other is frame aggregation technology in the MAC layer. Both the technologies of MIMO and frame aggregation enable the maximum data rate to attain 150Mbps in IEEE 802.11n [19].

In this chapter, we employ IEEE 802.11n as the WLAN implementation for in-hospital healthcare monitoring. In the following sections, we will present

Table 2. Information of IEEE 802.11 standards [18] (©2007 IEEE, reproduced with permission).

802.11 Protocol	Release	Frequency (GHz)	Maximum data rate (Mbps)	Modulation	Coverage (m) (indoor/outdoor)
–	Jun 1997	2.4	2	DSSS/FHSS	20/100
a	Sep 1999	3.7/5	54	OFDM	35/120
b	Sep 1999	2.4	11	DSSS	38/140
g	Jun 2003	2.4	54	OFDM/DSSS	38/140
n	Oct 2009	2.4/5	150	MIMO−OFDM	70/250

resource allocation in the IEEE 802.11n based WLAN for in-hospital healthcare monitoring.

2. Literature Review

In the physical layer of IEEE 802.11n, orthogonal frequency division multiplexing (OFDM) and multiple input multiple output (MIMO) are employed. OFDM efficiently resolves the problem of inter-symbol interference by transmitting multiple parallel low-rate streams instead of a single high-rate stream. MIMO can enhance the system capacity by using a number of transmit and receive antennas for spatial diversity [20]. MIMO-OFDM takes full advantage of both MIMO and OFDM technologies. It enables a WLAN to enhance its system capacity, to lower its bit error rate (BER), and to satisfy the quality of service (QOS) of network traffic.

The issues with respect to resource allocation in a 802.11n WLAN mainly include network scheduling and admission control [20]. Scheduling is a way to improve system performance by allocating system resource, involving the number of antennas for each user, the number of subcarriers for each antenna, and the amount of transmit power for each subcarrier, etc. [21–23]. Admission control is a mechanism to determine whether or not a new user is admitted into the network. Once a user arriving, a network coordinator will estimate the QOS requirements of this user and judge whether network resource is sufficient to satisfy these requirements. If the resource is available, then, this user is allowed for admission [24–26].

The abovementioned literature is relevant to resource allocation schemes in the WLAN for a general purpose. These schemes cannot be applied to the scenario of healthcare monitoring. This inappropriate application attributes to a few characteristics as follows. Firstly, the channels in hospital environment are different from those in general environment due to the effects of medical equipments and specificities of a hospital's physical layout. Additionally, the special channel characteristics in a hospital would lead to the types of imperfect CSI in a wireless healthcare system different from those in general environment. Finally, the electromagnetic interference (EMI) of wireless devices must be restricted below an acceptable level in a hospital to protect medical equipments. As a result, the transmit power in the WLAN should also be restricted to suppress the EMI on medical equipments. In the following, we review the literature on channel characteristics, on types of imperfect CSI, and on EMI in hospital environment.

2.1. Channel characteristics in hospital environments

Based on their measurement, Seong-Cheol et al. in [27] present a view that a line-of-sight (LOS) channel is well represented by the Rician model, while a non-line-of-sight (NLOS) channel is well represented by the Rayleigh model. This view is supported by [28–30] in various scenarios, such as closed corridors, open corridors, classrooms, and computer labs. The abovementioned research, however, does not focus on hospital environment, so those channel models cannot be directly applied to hospital environment.

To the best of our knowledge, Huang and Francisco in [31, 32] originally propose the WLAN channel models in hospital environment by measuring channel characteristics in a bedroom of Kempenhaeghe Hospital, Heeze, the Netherlands. Generally, each channel model proposed in [31] is composed of a large-scale fading model and a small-scale fading model. With respect to a particular channel model, its relevant parameters may be different from those in other models.

2.1.1. Large-scale fading model

It is shown in [31] that the large-scale fading model can be described as a log-distance fading model. The log-distance fading (dB) at distance d can be expressed as

$$F(d) = F(d_0) + 10n \log(d/d_0) \tag{1}$$

where $F(x)$ represent the large-scale fading at distance x; d_0 is the reference distance; n is the fading exponent.

2.1.2. Small-scale fading model

Huang and Francisco in [31] build a flat-fading model to describe the small-scaled fading, because the signal duration of most 2.4GHz systems is larger than the maximum delay spread [31]. Usually, the Rayleigh model, the Ricean model, or the Nakagami model are employed to represent a flat-fading model [33]. Additionally, the Rayleigh and Ricean models can be approximately viewed as special cases of Nakagami models. Specifically, assume that the probability density function (pdf) of fading A in a Nakagami distribution is

$$f(A) = \frac{2m^m A^{2m-1}}{\sigma^m \Gamma(m)} e^{-mA^2/\sigma} \tag{2}$$

where $\Gamma(.)$ is a Gamma function; σ and m are two parameters related to a Nakagami distribution.

Then, when $m = 1$, the Nakagami channel model can be simplified as a Rayleigh model; when $m = (K+1)^2/(2K+1)$, the Nakagami channel model can be approximately transformed into a Ricean model. Since Rayleigh and Ricean models are special cases of Nakagami models, the Nakagami channel model is widely used to represent flat-fading channels [34–36].

As for the channel models in hospital environment, Huang and Francisco in [31] take into account three LOS cases and one NLOS case. These three LOS cases include the transmission across the room (AR), the transmission along the front board of the bed (AB), and the transmission along the bedside (AS) [31]. Based on the measurement in [31], the NLOS case and the AB case can be modeled as Rayleigh models, while the AR and AS cases can be modeled as Ricean models. In view of the relationship between the Rayleigh or Ricean model and the Nakagami model, we can safely apply Nakagami models with different parameters to describe different channels in a hospital.

2.2. Imperfect CSI in WLAN

For resource allocation, the flow of channel state information (CSI) in a centralized network is shown in Fig.4 [37]. In this flow, three steps are taken for resource allocation in one time slot. The first step is *detecting CSI*. Specifically the central unit sends out pilots whose amplitudes are known by each user. Then each user estimates the channel characteristics by comparing the amplitudes o signals at the receive end and those at the transmit end. In the second step, each user sends the estimated CSI back to the central unit, and we call this step *CSI feedback*. The third step is *sending out decisions on resource allocation*. The central unit determines the allocation of resources among users based on their CSI feedback. Then, the decision of resource allocation is sent to each user.

Based on the information flow shown in Fig.4, there are mainly five types of imperfect CSI. We will discuss these types of imperfect CSI and their respective causes.

The first type of imperfect CSI is due to the errors of channel detection, that is, step one of Fig.4 [38]. We denote this type of imperfect CSI by *forward channel detection based imperfect CSI (ForCD-ICSI)*. In a noisy forward channel, the detected channel fading may not be the exact channel fading. Based on this inexact channel fading, the central unit cannot send the decisions on resource allocation to each user.

The second type of imperfect CSI is caused by the errors of CSI feedback, that is, step two of Fig.4 [39]. We call it *feedback based imperfect CSI (Fe-ICSI)*. In a noisy feedback channel, the detected channel fading may be different from the exact channel fading. Thus, the central unit cannot get the exact CSI feedback from each user. If the automatic repeat request (ARQ) is used in upper layers, the Fe-ICSI would lead to a feedback delay. When the feedback delay is larger than a time slot for resource allocation, the central unit cannot access the CSI in current time slot. This delay would cause inefficiency of resource allocation.

The third type of imperfect CSI is owing to the lossy compression of CSI at the user end [37], and we call it *feedback compression based imperfect CSI (FC-ICSI)*. Subject to limited feedback bandwidth and acceptable feedback delay,

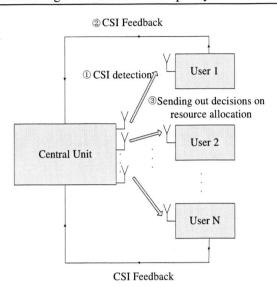

Figure 4. Information flow of a centralized network [37] (©2008 IEEE, reproduced with permission).

users prefer to employ as few bits as possible to send the feedback CSI [40]. Specifically, they would quantize the detected CSI at the user end before sending it to the central unit. Therefore, a loss of CSI occurs when signals arrive at the central unit.

The fourth type of imperfect CSI depends on the variation of channel characteristics and the feedback delay [40]. We call it *fast-fading channel based imperfect CSI (FF-ICSI)*. Caused by the doppler effect, channel fading would vary fast. Owing to the delay of transmission and estimation, the CSI would not be estimated at the receive end before it varies at the transmit end. Thus, the central unit cannot allocate resource based on the up-to-date CSI.

The fifth type of imperfect CSI is related to duplexing schemes utilized in a system. If this system uses the frequency division duplexing (FDD) scheme, the data transmission on the forward channel and that on the feedback channel would work at different frequency bands [41]. In this case, the CSI estimated at the user end cannot be applied to the transmission from users to the central unit.

We call this type of imperfect CSI as *FDD based imperfect CSI (FDD-ICSI)*.

In general, we should take into account the five types of imperfect CSI when using CSI to allocate resource. As for the specific case of healthcare monitoring, we only need to consider the first three types. The reasons are as follows: the FF-ICSI depends on Doppler effects, which are caused by the relative mobility of transmitters and receivers. However, in a hospital, patients and clinicians can only move at a low speed, and in this case, the Doppler effect can be neglected [31]. Therefore, the fourth type of imperfect CSI, FF-ICSI, can be ignored in our analysis. As for the fifth type of imperfect CSI, FDD-ICSI, we can also neglect it, since a WLAN usually employs time division duplexing (TDD) instead of FDD [42].

2.3. Electromagnetic interference in medical equipments

Until now, research on EMI in hospital environment has primarily focused on the immunity to mobile phones. Tan et al. in [43] state that some medical equipments are sensitive to the EMI of cellular phones. These equipments include ventilators, infusion pumps, and ECG monitors. Then, a test on EMI susceptibility is carried by the Medicines and Healthcare Products Regulatory Agency (MHRA) of U.K. [44]. By measuring the EMI of both mobile phones and personal communication networks, researchers show that external pacemakers, anesthesia machines, respirators, defibrillators are also susceptible to EMI. Trigano et al. in [45] and Calcagnini et al. in [46] study the EMI of GSM mobile phones on pacemakers and that on infusion pumps, respectively. Their study results show that infusion pumps and pacemakers would be inhibited by the EMI of GSM mobile phones. With the implementation of 3G mobile phone systems in the United States, Japan, Hong Kong etc., some standards about EMI in the 3G band are proposed [47–49]. In 2007, the EN60601-1-2 standard is published by the International Electrotechnical Committee (IEC). In this standard, the acceptable levels of EMI are recommended as below 3V/m and 10V/m for nonlife-support medical equipments and life-support medical equipments, respectively. In view of the advances of electromagnetic compatibility (EMC) technologies, some hospitals in Singapore and the U.K. relax the EMI level recommended in the EN60601-1-2 standard, and mobile phones are permitted to use in some areas of hospitals [50]. Chi-Kit et al. in [51] perform a EMI test in view of the EMC of medical equipments. The results of this test show that ECG monitors, radiographic systems, audio evoked potential systems, and ultrasonic fetal heart detectors are sensitive to EMI [51]. Based on the previous research, we can summarize that the medical equipments possibly sensitive to the EMI of cellular phones include fetal monitors, infusion pumps, syringe pumps, ECG monitors, external pacemakers, respirators, anesthesia machines, and defibrillators [52].

The abovementioned literature focuses on the EMI of mobile phones. However, the policies of using mobile phones in a hospital may not be applied to the scenario of wireless healthcare [53], because clinicians and patients use wireless devices to transmit data for healthcare monitoring. Only lowering transmit power of a patient device may reduce the QoS of data transmission and lead to the risk of data loss. To tradeoff between transmit power restriction and Qos requirements, Phond in [54] propose a EMI-aware scheme to design the system for healthcare monitoring. In this scheme, a network coordinator adjusts the transmit power of patient devices based on the utilization of medical equipments. A device is required to lower transmit power if its neighbouring medical equipments are turned on and otherwise required to enhance transmit power.

3. Resource allocation in wireless healthcare systems

In this section, we would discuss the issue of resource allocation in a wireless healthcare system. Firstly, we build up a model to solve the problem of resource allocation with perfect CSI and without EMI constraints. This model can be viewed as a benchmark for the following cases. Next, we take into account the EMI constraints as well as imperfect CSI for resource allocation.

3.1. Resource allocation with perfect CSI and without EMI constraints

In this section, we first introduce the general background of resource allocation for healthcare monitoring, including the architecture of an in-hospital monitoring system and the types of traffic in this system. Then, we discuss the issues of optimal bandwidth allocation with perfect CSI and without EMI constraints.

3.1.1. General background of resource allocation

From the perspective of coverage, healthcare monitoring systems can mainly be classified into two types: in-hospital monitoring systems [9,55,56] and remote monitoring systems [2,20,57,58]. In-hospital monitoring systems are mainly to serve inpatients who need intensive monitoring, such as the patients staying in emergent room (ER) for treatments. Once an emergent condition occurs, healthcare staff must be alerted, since a delay of even a few seconds could sometimes mean a loss of life. Remote monitoring systems are mainly to serve chronic or elderly patients, and emergent conditions do not occur as frequently as in in-hospital monitoring systems.

As shown in Fig. 3, a WLAN covers the area from patient beds to the monitoring center, and it is for data transmission from patient computing devices to the monitoring center. Due to the limited ability of decision making in patient devices, medical data need to be sent to the monitoring center for more detailed diagnosis. According to the status of patients, the data sent from different devices may have different acceptable delays and should be given different priorities. Additionally, when an abnormal status is detected, a communication via video conferences will start between patients and clinicians staying at the monitoring center [13]. Finally, some messages on patient information should be transmitted to the monitoring center. Thus, we take into account here a traffic in the WLAN mainly including messages, video conferences, and medical data with different priorities. In the traditional scheme, all the subcarriers of WLAN are allocated among a message part, an application part and a data part [13]. The message part is for the transmission of messages; the application part is for video conferences; the data part is for the transmission of medical data. This traditional scheme would cause the application part to be underutilized, since video conferences occur infrequently. The underutilization of bandwidth would lower the capacity of patients in the WLAN for in-hospital healthcare monitoring.

A dynamic data transmission scheme is proposed in [16] to enhance the capacity of patients supported by the WLAN for in-hospital healthcare monitoring. In this scheme, the application part is used for the transmission of medical data when some subcarriers for video conference are idle. If all subcarriers are busy, we can store medical data in patient devices. Otherwise, we can free the memory of devices by transmitting the stored medical data to the monitoring

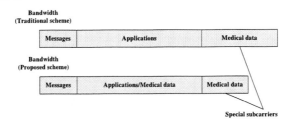

Figure 5. Proposed scheme of bandwidth allocation [16] (©2010 IEEE, reproduced with permission).

center. If both the memory size of a patient device and the acceptable delay for data transmission are unlimited, then, we do not need to use extra subcarriers for the transmission of medical data. However, in reality, both the memory size of a patient device and the acceptable delay are limited. Thus, some extra subcarriers specially to transmit medical data are required even with the proposed scheme, but the proposed scheme can save subcarriers in comparison with the traditional scheme. Fig.5 shows both the traditional scheme and the proposed scheme.

3.1.2.   Optimal bandwidth allocation with perfect CSI and without EMI constraints

Patient status can be classified into 'high-degree (H)', 'low-degree (L)', and 'normal (N)'. They represent different emergency degrees of patient status [59]. According to their corresponding patient status, medical data may have different priorities. Medical data with a high priority would have a smaller acceptable delay. Based on the scheme to transmit medical data, we discuss how to maximize the network patient capacity, which is defined as the capacity of patients supported by the WLAN subject to its maximal potential number of subcarriers.

We note that N_u is the number of patients; and N_T is the number of time slots during monitoring. The objective of maximizing the network patient capacity is shown as equation (3a) below. As presented in Section 3.1, a patient device would collect data from medical sensors and temporarily store these data into this device's memory to make decisions on patient status. For each patient device, the amount of data in the memory is the same as that in time slot $k-1$ plus the new data arrival, minus the data sent in slot k (shown as equation (3b)). Of course, the amount of data stored in a patient device's memory should not exceed the memory size to avoid data loss (shown as equation (3c)). In equation (3b) and equation (3c), $M_i^{(k)}[bits]$ denotes the amount of data in the memory of the ith patient device in the kth time slot; $B_i^{(k)}[Hz]$ denotes the bandwidth allocated to the ith device in the kth time slot; $\eta_i^{(k)}[bps/Hz]$ denotes the bandwidth efficiency available to the ith device in the kth time slot; $a_i^{(k)}[bps]$ denotes the data arrival rate of the ith device in the kth time slot; $T_c[s]$ is the duration of one time slot; $M_i^{\max}[bits]$ denotes the memory size of the ith device. Additionally, the total amount of bandwidth in the kth time slot, both for applications and for data transmission, equals the total amount of bandwidth in the $(k-1)$th time slot plus the additional amount of bandwidth (of special subcarriers) in the kth time slot (shown as equation (3d)). The total amount of bandwidth allocated should not exceed the overall WLAN bandwidth available (shown as equation (3e)). In equation (3d) and equation (3e), $B_a^{(k)}[Hz]$ denotes the bandwidth for applications in the kth time slot; $B_{total}[Hz]$ denotes the total amount of bandwidth; $\Delta B[Hz]$ denotes the bandwidth of one subcarrier; $S^{(k)}$ denotes the number of special subcarriers in the kth ($k = 1, 2 \cdots N_T$) time slot. According to different patient status, the acceptable delays for data transmission are also different. Let $\Delta T_1[s]$, $\Delta T_2[s]$, and $\Delta T_3[s]$ be the acceptable delays of data transmission when the patient status is 'H', 'L', and 'N', respectively. For simplicity, we assume that the acceptable delay to transmit data in state 'N' is infinite, that is, $\Delta T_3 = \infty$. Then, to meet their respective delay requirements, the transmission of data in states 'H' and 'L' should meet equation (3f) and equation (3g).

Building on the aforementioned analysis, the problem of maximizing network patient capacity can be described as a dynamic programming problem, and this programming problem in the kth ($k = 1, 2 \cdots N_T$) time slot can be expressed as

$$\max_{B_i^{(k)}} N_u \tag{3a}$$

$$\text{s.t. } M_i^{(k)} = \max\left\{ (a_i^{(k)} - \eta_i^{(k)} B_i^{(k)})T_c + M_i^{(k-1)}, 0 \right\}, \forall i \tag{3b}$$

$$M_i^{(k)} \leq M_i^{\max}, \forall i \tag{3c}$$

$$\sum_{i=1}^{N_u} B_i^{(k)} + B_a^{(k)} = S^{(k)} \Delta B + \sum_{i=1}^{N_u} B_i^{(k-1)} \tag{3d}$$

$$\sum_{i=1}^{N_u} B_i^{(k)} + B_a^{(k)} \leq B_{total} \tag{3e}$$

$$a_i^{(k)} T_c \leq \eta_i^{(k)} B_i^{(k)} \Delta T_1 \quad (i \in \mathbf{H}) \tag{3f}$$

$$a_i^{(k)} T_c \leq \eta_i^{(k)} B_i^{(k)} \Delta T_2 \quad (i \in \mathbf{L}) \tag{3g}$$

3.2. Optimal bandwidth allocation in view of EMI

In a wireless healthcare system, both patients and healthcare staff would employ devices to communicate or send patient's medical data. Both the patient devices and healthcare staff devices would cause EMI to other devices and medical equipments. The medical equipments in a hospital can mainly be classified into life-support equipments and non-life-support equipments. While a life-support equipment (e.g., a blood pressure monitor or an infusion pump) is used to sustain the life of patients who are critically ill or injured, a non-life-support equipment (e.g., a defibrillator) routinely collects some medical data of patients [54]. Medical equipments never cause EMI to other equipments or devices.

To analyze EMI on medical equipments, we need to employ a basic relationship between radiated power $P(W)$ and electric field $E(V/m)$, that is, $E = Z\sqrt{P}/D$. $Z(\Omega)$ is the impedance of free space. $D(m)$ is the distance between the transmitter and the receiver. The relationship between radiated power $P(W)$ and electric field $E(V/m)$ is recommended by IEC [60] as $E = 7\sqrt{P}/D$ and $E = 23\sqrt{P}/D$ for a non-life-support equipment and a life-support equipment, respectively. For a medical equipment, the summation of all potential EMI should be less than an acceptable level of EMI. If we use $E_{NLS}(p)$ and $E_{LS}(q)$ to represent this EMI level for a non-life-support equipment p and a life-support equipment q, respectively, then, we have

$$\sum_{A=1}^{A_t} \frac{7\sqrt{P_{NLS}(A)}}{D_{NLS}(A)} + \sum_{x=1}^{X_t} \frac{7\sqrt{P_t(x)}}{D_x(p)} \leq E_{NLS}(p) \tag{4}$$

$$\sum_{A=1}^{A_t} \frac{23\sqrt{P_{LS}(A)}}{D_{LS}(A)} + \sum_{x=1}^{X_t} \frac{23\sqrt{P_t(x)}}{D_x(q)} \leq E_{LS}(q) \tag{5}$$

where $P_{NLS}(A)$ and $P_{LS}(A)$ are the maximal potential transmit power of a healthcare staff A to satisfy the EMI requirement of a non-life-support equipment and a life-support equipment, respectively; $D_{NLS}(A)$ and $D_{LS}(A)$ are the distances from the healthcare staff device to the non-life-support device equipment A and the life-supporting device equipment A, respectively; $P_t(x)$ is transmit power of a patient device x; $D_x(p)$ and $D_x(q)$ are the distances between the transmitter of the device x and the non-life-support p or the life-support equipment q; X_t and A_t are the number of patient devices and healthcare staff devices being turned on.

In a real hospital environment, healthcare staff devices, patient devices, life-support medical equipments, and non-life-support medical equipments may operate at the same time. Thus, the transmit power of both a healthcare staff device and a patient device should meet equation (4) as well as equation (5) to avoid unacceptable EMI on medical equipments. If we denote the maximal transmit power at time slot k for patient device i by $P_{max}^{(k)}(i)$, then, $P_{max}^{(k)}(i)$ should be the maximum of device i's transmit power that satisfies both equation (4) and equation (5).

Based on the aforementioned analysis, the problem of maximizing network patient capacity can be transformed into a dynamic programming problem subject to the maximal transmit power of patient devices. This dynamic programming problem has the same objective to equation (3a)), and its first six constraints are also the same to equations ((3b)-(3g)). In addition, the problem in view of EMI have three more constraints. Each patient device has its own limit of transmit power to avoid unacceptable EMI on medical equipments, shown in equation (6a)). Given the transmit power of a patient device, the signal to noise ratio (SNR) and bandwidth efficiency are represented by equation (6b)) and equation (6c)), respectively.

$$P_i^{(k)} \leq P_{max}^{(k)}(i), \forall i \tag{6a}$$

$$r_i^{(k)} = P_i^{(k)} \left| h_i^{(k)} \right|^2 \Big/ \left(B_i^{(k)} \sigma^2 \right), \forall i \tag{6b}$$

$$\eta_i^{(k)} = \left[\sum_{p=1}^{m} \exp\{p/r_i^k\} \sum_{l=n-m}^{(n+m-2p)p} a_{p,l} \right.$$
$$\left. \times \sum_{j=1}^{l+1} E_{l+2-j}\left(p/r_i^k\right) \right]_i^{(k)}, \forall i \tag{6c}$$

where $\eta_i^{(k)}$ is the bandwidth efficiency for patient device i at time slot k; $P_i^{(k)}[W]$ is the transmit power of patient device i at time slot k; $\sigma^2[W/Hz]$ is the noise spectral density; $r_i^{(k)}$ is the signal to noise ratio (SNR) for patient device i at time slot k; $h_i^{(k)}$ is the channel fading for patient device i at time slot k; $a_{p,l}$ is a coefficient depending on the characteristics of MIMO channels [61]; $E_l(x)$ is the l-order exponential integral function of x, and $E_l(x) = \int_1^\infty e^{-xt} t^{-l} dt$; $f\left(\sigma_e^2; r\right) = r/\left((1 + \sigma_e^2)(1 + \sigma_e^2(1 + r))\right)$.

3.3. Optimal bandwidth allocation with imperfect CSI

In the scenario of imperfect CSI, all the parameters of this programming problem are the same as those in equation (3) except the bandwidth efficiency. Specifically, the bandwidth efficiency in case of imperfect CSI is an estimated bandwidth efficiency instead of an exact bandwidth efficiency, and the details of estimation process are addressed in [62]. We denote the estimated bandwidth efficiency as $\overline{\eta}_i^{(k)}[bps/Hz]$. Then, in the kth time slot, the problem for resource allocation can be described as

$$
\begin{aligned}
Max \quad & N_u \\
s.t. \quad & M_i^{(k)} = Max\left\{(a_i^{(k)} - \overline{\eta}_i^{(k)} B_i^{(k)})T_c + M_i^{(k-1)}, 0\right\} \\
& M_i^{(k)} \leq M_i^{\max} \\
& \sum_{i=1}^{N_u} B_i^{(k)} + B_a^{(k)} = S^{(k)} \Delta B + \sum_{i=1}^{N_u} B_i^{(k-1)} \qquad (7) \\
& \sum_{i=1}^{N_u} B_i^{(k)} + B_a^{(k)} \leq B_{total} \\
& a_i^{(k)} T_c \leq \overline{\eta}_i^{(k)} B_i^{(k)} \Delta T_1 \quad (i \in \mathbf{H}) \\
& a_i^{(k)} T_c \leq \overline{\eta}_i^{(k)} B_i^{(k)} \Delta T_2 \quad (i \in \mathbf{L})
\end{aligned}
$$

As for the $\overline{\eta}_i^{(k)}$ in equation (7), we should take into account the first three types of imperfect CSI presented in Section 2.2, namely, ForCD-ICSI, Fe-ICSI, and FC-ICSI. For simplicity, we denote ForCD-ICSI, Fe-ICSI, and FC-ICSI by type I, type II, and type III imperfect CSI, respectively.

3.3.1. Effect of type I imperfect CSI

Type I imperfect CSI is caused by estimation error, which is usually modeled as a complex circular Gaussian random variable [62]. Based on this model, the estimation of bandwidth efficiency $\bar{\eta}_i^{(k)}$ in the MIMO-OFDM based WLAN can be denoted as equation (8) [61].

$$\bar{\eta}_i^{(k)} = \left[\sum_{p=1}^m \exp\{p/f\left(\sigma_e^2;r\right)\} \sum_{l=n-m}^{(n+m-2p)p} a_{p,l} \right.$$
$$\left. \times \sum_{j=1}^{l+1} E_{l+2-j}\left(p/f\left(\sigma_e^2;r\right)\right) \right]_i^{(k)} \quad (8)$$

where $[x]_i^{(k)}$ shows that the value of bandwidth efficiency is x for the ith user in the kth time slot; n_T and n_R are the number of transit antennas and receive antennas, respectively; $m = \min\{n_T, n_R\}$ and $n = \max\{n_T, n_R\}$; $a_{p,l}$ is a coefficient depending on the characteristics of MIMO channels [61]; r is the average signal-to-noise ratio for data transmission; σ_e^2 is the variance of estimation error; $E_l(x)$ is the l-order exponential integral function of x, and $E_l(x) = \int_1^\infty e^{-xt} t^{-l} dt$; $f\left(\sigma_e^2;r\right) = r/\left((1+\sigma_e^2)(1+\sigma_e^2(1+r))\right)$.

3.3.2. Effect of type II imperfect CSI

Type II imperfect CSI is due to the error of CSI feedback. The $\bar{\eta}_i^{(k)}$ can be expressed as

$$\bar{\eta}_i^{(k)} = \begin{cases} \eta_i^{(k)} & \text{Successful CSI feedback} \\ \eta_0 & \text{Unsuccessful CSI feedback} \end{cases} \quad (9)$$

where η_0 is a predefined bandwidth efficiency as the CSI transmission failed in feedback. If we denote the probability of a successful CSI feedback as p_e and use ARQ schemes with M retransmission at most in upper layers, then, the $\bar{\eta}_i^{(k)}$ can be alternatively expressed as

$$\bar{\eta}_i^{(k)} = \begin{cases} \eta_i^{(k)} & \text{with a probability of } 1 - (p_e)^M \\ \eta_0 & \text{with a probability of } (p_e)^M \end{cases} \quad (10)$$

3.3.3. Effect of type III imperfect CSI

Type III imperfect CSI is caused by quantization errors. The bandwidth efficiency estimated in the feedback is usually quantized for a smaller number of information bits. Thus, the estimated bandwidth efficiency is not the exact bandwidth efficiency. Mathematically, the $\overline{\eta}_i^{(k)}$ can be represented as

$$\overline{\eta}_i^{(k)} = \left[\eta_i^{(k)}\right]_l \tag{11}$$

where $\eta_i^{(k)}$ is the exact bandwidth efficiency; $[x]_l$ shows that l bits are used to represent x in the feedback. For example, assuming $\eta_i^{(k)} \in [0, 1]$, we divide the section $[0, 1]$ into 2^l parts and use $m/2^l$ $(m = 0 \cdots 2^l - 1)$ to estimate x, when x falls into the mth part.

3.3.4. Effects of type I, II and III imperfect CSI

In view of equation (8), equation (9), equation (10), and equation (11), the overall $\overline{\eta}_i^{(k)}$ can be denoted as equation (12).

$$\overline{\eta}_i^{(k)} = \begin{cases} \eta_0 & \text{with } (p_e)^M \\ \left[\left[\sum_{p=1}^{m} \exp\{p/f\left(\sigma_e^2; r\right)\} \sum_{l=n-m}^{(n+m-2p)p} a_{p,l} \right. \\ \left. \times \sum_{j=1}^{l+1} E_{l+2-j}\left(p/f\left(\sigma_e^2; r\right)\right)\right]_l\right]_i^{(k)} \\ & \text{with } 1 - (p_e)^M \end{cases} \tag{12}$$

3.4.   Simulation and results

In this section, we discuss the simulation results based on the analysis in Section 3.1-3.3. Firstly, we demonstrate the effects of imperfect CSI on system performance. Then, we discuss network patient capacity with both the proposed scheme and the traditional scheme in view of imperfect CSI and EMI constraints. Finally, we discuss the data loss and data unavailability due to imperfect CSI.

3.4.1.   Effects of imperfect CSI on system performance

In this section, we present the potential effects of each type of imperfect CSI. According to equation (8), the type I imperfect CSI will underestimate bandwidth efficiency and overestimate the number of subcarriers to support data transmission in the whole system. Then, the network patient capacity would decrease in the system, given the maximal potential number of subcarriers.

According to equation (10), ARQ schemes with M retransmission at most are employed in upper layers. After M retransmission, η_0 is used to estimate bandwidth efficiency, and it is not the exact bandwidth efficiency. If η_0 underestimates the exact bandwidth efficiency, the transmission of medical data could succeed at a cost of lower network patient capacity. If η_0 overestimates the exact bandwidth efficiency, then, the transmission of medical data would fail, and data can only be stored in patient devices. When one data transmission fails, two results may occur: one is that medical data cannot be transmitted to the monitoring center within their acceptable delays and we call this case *data unavailability*; the other is that the medical data would be lost and the data loss occurs when the patient devices are filled up. Therefore, in the following simulations, we discuss data loss, data unavailability as well as change of number of subcarriers caused by the type II imperfect CSI.

According to equation (11), the type III imperfect CSI would underestimate bandwidth efficiency, since the estimated bandwidth efficiency is quantified as the left point of a quantification interval. The underestimation of bandwidth efficiency would not lead to data loss or data unavailability, but it would lower the network patient capacity.

In view of the effects of all types of imperfect CSI, we will discuss the network patient capacity in Section 3.4.2. Then, we will discuss the data loss and data unavailability due to type II imperfect CSI in Section 3.4.3.

3.4.2. Network patient capacity

The parameters in the simulation are in the following: $N_T = 50000$, T_c=0.1s, $\Delta T_1 = 0.5T_c$, $\Delta T_2 = T_c$, ΔB=0.8MHz, $a_i^{(k)}$=800kbps, the maximal potential number of retransmissions M=2, P_e=0.1, r=10dB, p=0.8. The network patient capacity is illustrated in Fig.6. Fig.6 shows that the proposed scheme can enhance the network patient capacity in comparison with the traditional scheme. In addition, the patient capacity decreases with p in both the proposed scheme and the traditional scheme. Finally, both the imperfect CSI and EMI constraints would lower the network patient capacity.

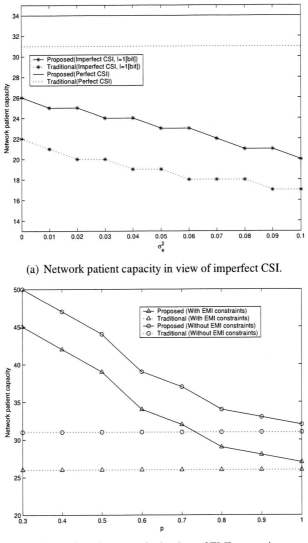

(a) Network patient capacity in view of imperfect CSI.

(b) Network patient capacity in view of EMI constraints.

Figure 6. Network patient capacity.

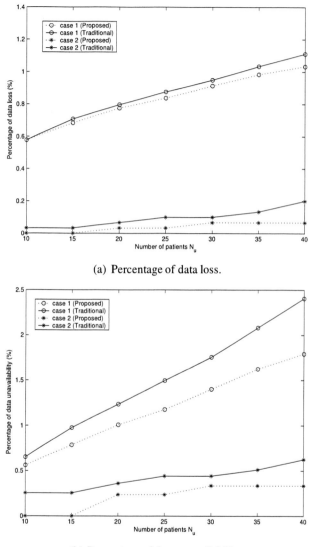

(a) Percentage of data loss.

(b) Percentage of data unavailability.

Figure 7. Percentage of data loss and data unavailability vs. number of patients.

3.4.3. Data loss and data unavailability due to imperfect CSI

As mentioned in Section 3.4.1, type II imperfect CSI may lead to data loss and data unavailability. In the following, we discuss both data loss and data unavailability through two cases. In the first case, we only take into account type II imperfect CSI. This case does not exist in reality, and it is only viewed as a benchmark for the following case. In the second case, we consider all three types of imperfect CSI.

The percentage of data loss and that of data unavailability are illustrated in Fig.7(a) and Fig.7(b), respectively. Fig.7 shows that the proposed scheme can attain a smaller data loss and data unavailability than the traditional scheme in both cases. Fig.7 also shows that the data loss and data unavailability would increase with the rise of η_0. In addition, the data loss and data unavailability in case 1 may attain above 0.5% as $\eta_0 = 10$, but for the same η_0, the data loss and data unavailability in case 2 is below 0.5%. In other words, both the data loss and data unavailability are mitigated by the combination of three types of imperfect CSI in case 2.

4. Conclusion

This chapter is devoted to studying the network patient capacity in a wireless healthcare monitoring system. To enhance the network patient capacity, we propose a novel scheme for bandwidth allocation in a WLAN. In this scheme, we take into account both the imperfect CSI and EMI constraints. As for imperfect CSI, we consider three types of imperfect CSI for healthcare monitoring. Then, we compare the network patient capacity with our proposed scheme and that with the traditional scheme. For all scenarios with respect to EMI constraints and three types of imperfect CSI, we conclude that our proposed scheme could attain a larger network patient capacity than the traditional scheme, given the acceptable data loss and data unavailability,.

With the proposed scheme, we can estimate the network patient capacity that one WLAN deployment can support. If this capacity is exceeded by the actual number of patients in a hospital, then the network would need to use more parallel WLAN deployment until the number of WLAN deployment attain the maximal potential number in a hospital. Therefore, by enhancing the network patient capacity of one WLAN deployment, we equally enhance the maximal number of patients in the whole system. This study can help in dimensioning the network and enhancing network performance for the design of wireless healthcare monitoring systems.

Acknowledgements

Parts of this work were supported by the Natural Sciences and Engineering Research Council (NSERC) and industrial and government partners, through the Healthcare Support through Information Technology Enhancements (hSITE) Strategic Research Network; and parts were supported by the Fonds Québécois de Recherche sur la Nature et les Technologies (FQRNT).

References

[1] WHO (1998): Life in the 21st century - a vision for all - fifty facts from the world health report.

[2] Rashvand, H. F., V. T. Salcedo, et al. (2008). "Ubiquitous wireless telemedicine." IET Communications, 2(2): 237-254.

[3] Dowler, N. and Hall, C.J. (1995). "Safety issues in telesurgery -summary." IEE Colloquium on 'Towards Telesugery'.

[4] Choi, Y. B., J. S. Krause, et al. (2006). "Telemedicine in the USA: standardization through information management and technical applications." IEEE Communications Magazine, 44(4): 41-48.

[5] Istepanian, R. S. H., E. Jovanov, et al. (2004). "Guest Editorial Introduction to the Special Section on M-Health: Beyond Seamless Mobility and Global Wireless Health-Care Connectivity." IEEE Transactions on Information Technology in Biomedicine, 8(4): 405-414.

[6] Sneha, S. and U. Varshney (2009). "Enabling ubiquitous patient monitoring: Model, decision protocols, opportunities and challenges." Decis. Support Syst, 46(3): 606-619.

[7] S.E.Kern, D. Jaron. (2003). "Healthcare technology, economics and policy: an evolving balance." IEEE Engineering in Medicine and Biology Magazine, 22(1): 16-19.

[8] Vasilakos, A. V., C. Hsiao-Hwa, et al. (2009). "Guest editorial wireless and pervasive communications for healthcare." IEEE Journal on Selected Areas in Communications, 27(4): 361-364.

[9] Golmie, N., D. Cypher, et al. (2005). "Performance analysis of low rate wireless technologies for medical applications." Computer Communications, 28(10): 1266-1275.

[10] Varshney, U. and S. Sneha (2006). "Patient monitoring using ad hoc wireless networks: reliability and power management." IEEE Communications Magazine, 44(4): 49-55.

[11] Varshney, U. (2008). "A framework for supporting emergency messages in wireless patient monitoring." Decision Support Systems, 45(4): 981-996.

[12] Sneha, S. and U. Varshney (2009). "Enabling ubiquitous patient monitoring: Model, decision protocols, opportunities and challenges." Decision Support Systems, 46(3): 606-619.

[13] Vergados, D. J., D. D. Vergados, et al. (2006). "NGL03-6: Applying Wireless DiffServ for QoS Provisioning in Mobile Emergency Telemedicine." IEEE Global Telecommunications Conference.

[14] Cypher, D., N. Chevrollier, et al. (2006). "Prevailing over wires in healthcare environments: benefits and challenges." IEEE Communications Magazine, 44(4): 56-63.

[15] Yifan, C., T. Jianqi, et al. (2009). "Cooperative Communications in Ultra-Wideband Wireless Body Area Networks: Channel Modeling and System Diversity Analysis." IEEE Journal on Selected Areas in Communications, 27(1): 5-16.

[16] Di Lin, Fabrice Labeau (2010). "A scheme of bandwidth allocation for the transmission of medical data." 44th IEEE Asilomar Conference on Signals, Systems, and Computers.

[17] Varshney, U. (2006). "Using wireless technologies in healthcare." Int. J. Mob. Commun, 4(3): 354-368.

[18] "IEEE 802.11: Wireless LAN Medium Access Control (MAC) and Physical Layer (PHY) Specifications (2007 revision)." IEEE-SA. 12 June 2007. doi:10.1109/IEEESTD.2007.373646.

[19] "IEEE 802.11n-2009-Amendment 5: Enhancements for Higher Throughput." IEEE-SA. 29 October 2009. doi:10.1109/IEEESTD.2009.5307322.

[20] Niyato, D. and E. Hossain (2007). "Radio Resource Management in MIMO-OFDM- Mesh Networks: Issues and Approaches." IEEE Communications Magazine, 45(11): 100-107.

[21] Quentin H. Spencer, A. L. S., Martin Haardt (2004). "Zero-Forcing Methods for Downlink Spatial Multiplexing in Multiuser MIMO Channels." IEEE transactions on signal processing, 52(2): 461-471.

[22] Letaief, K. B. and Z. Ying Jun (2006). "Dynamic multiuser resource allocation and adaptation for wireless systems." IEEE Wireless Communications, 13(4): 38-47.

[23] Ho, W. W. L. and L. Ying-Chang (2009). "Optimal Resource Allocation for Multiuser MIMO-OFDM Systems With User Rate Constraints." IEEE Transactions on Vehicular Technology, 58(3): 1190-1203.

[24] Q. Liu, S. Zhou, and G. B. Giannakis (2005). "Queuing with Adaptive Modulation and Coding over Wireless Links: Cross-Layer Analysis and Design," IEEE Trans. Wireless Commun., 4(3): 1142-1153.

[25] Y. J. Zhang and K. B. Letaief (2006). "Cross-layer Adaptive Resource Management for Wireless Packet Networks with OFDM Signal," IEEE Trans. Wireless Commun, 5(11): 3244-3254.

[26] M. Chiang et al. (2005). "Balancing Transport and Physical Layers In Wireless Multihop Networks: Jointly Optimal Congestion Control and Power Control," IEEE JSAC, 23(1): 104-116.

[27] Seong-Cheol, K., H. L. Bertoni, et al. (1996). "Pulse propagation characteristics at 2.4 GHz inside buildings." IEEE Transactions on Vehicular Technology, 45(3): 579-592.

[28] Walker, E., H. J. Zepernick, et al. (1998). "Fading measurements at 2.4 GHz for the indoor radio propagation channel." International Zurich Seminar on Broadband Communications.

[29] Zepernick, H. J. and T. A. Wysocki (1999). "Multipath channel parameters for the indoor radio at 2.4 GHz ISM band." IEEE Vehicular Technology Conference.

[30] Robert Akl, D. T., Xinrong Li (2006). "Indoor propagation modeling at 2.4 GHZ for IEEE 802.11 networks." The sixth international multi-conference on wireless and optical communications networks and emerging technologies.

[31] L. Huang, R. d. F., and G. Dolmans (2009). "Channel measurement and modeling in medical environments." Third International Symposium on Medical Information and Communication Technology. Montreal, Canada.

[32] de Francisco, R., H. Li, et al. (2009). "Coexistence of WBAN and WLAN in Medical Environments." IEEE Vehicular Technology Conference.

[33] T. S. Rappaport (1996). "Wireless communications: principle & practice." Prentice Hall, Upper Saddle River, NJ.

[34] Li-Chun, W., L. Ya-Wen, et al. (2004). "Cross-layer goodput analysis for rate adaptive IEEE 802.11a WLAN in the generalized Nakagami fading channel." IEEE International Conference on Communications.

[35] Li-Chun, W., Y. Kuang-Nan, et al. (2006). "Joint rate and power adaptation for wireless local area networks in Nakagami fading channels." IEEE Wireless Communications and Networking Conference.

[36] Li-Chun, W., L. Wei-Cheng, et al. (2009). "Joint Rate and Power Adaptation for Wireless Local Area Networks in Generalized Nakagami Fading Channels." IEEE Transactions on Vehicular Technology, 58(3): 1375-1386.

[37] Love, D. J., R. W. Heath, et al. (2008). "An overview of limited feedback in wireless communication systems." IEEE Journal on Selected Areas in Communications, 26(8): 1341-1365.

[38] Ahmed, W. K. M. and P. J. McLane (2000). "Random coding error exponents for flat fading channels with realistic channel estimation." IEEE Journal on Selected Areas in Communications, 18(3): 369-379.

[39] Ekpenyong, A. E. and Y. F. Huang (2007). "Feedback Constraints for Adaptive Transmission." IEEE Signal Processing Magazine, 24(3): 69-78.

[40] Eriksson, T. and T. Ottosson (2007). "Compression of Feedback for Adaptive Transmission and Scheduling." Proceedings of the IEEE, 95(12): 2314-2321.

[41] Ekpenyong, A. E. and H. Yih-Fang (2006). "Feedback-detection strategies for adaptive modulation systems." IEEE Transactions on Communications, 54(10): 1735-1740.

[42] Kuhn, M., Ettefagh, A., Hammerstrom, I., Wittneben, A. (2006) "Two-way Communication for IEEE 802.11n WLANs Using Decode and Forward Relays." Fortieth Asilomar Conference on Signals, Systems and Computers.

[43] K.-S. Tan and I. Hinberg. (1994). "Radiofrequency susceptibility tests on medical equipment." IEEE 16th Annu. Int. Conf, 2: 998-999.

[44] "Electromagnetic compatibility of medical devices with mobile communications." in Medical Devices Bulletin DB9702. London, U.K.: Medical Devices Agency, 1997.

[45] A. J. Trigano, A. Azoulay,M. Rochdi, and A. Campillo. "Electromagnetic interference of external pacemakers by walkie-talkies and digital cellular phones: experimental study." Pacing Clin. Electrophysiol, 22(4): 588-593.

[46] G. Calcagnini, P. Bartolini, M. Floris, M. Triventi, P. Cianfanelli, G. Scavino, L. Proietti, and V. Barbaro. "Electromagnetic interference to infusion pumps from GSM mobile phones." IEEE 26th Annu. Int. Conf, 2: 3515-3518.

[47] Y. Chu and A. Ganz. (2004). "A mobile teletrauma system using 3G networks." IEEE Trans. Inf. Technol. Biomed, 8(4): 456-462.

[48] K. A. Banitsas, K. Perakis, S. Tachakra, and D. Koutsouris. "Use of 3G mobile phone links for teleconsultation between a moving ambulance and a hospital base station." J. Telemed. Telecare, 12(1): 23-26.

[49] E. A. V. Navarro, J. R.Mas, J. F. Navajas, and C. P. Alcega. "Performance of a 3G-based mobile telemedicine system." IEEE 3rd Consum. Commun. Netw. Conf, 2: 1023-1027.

[50] E-Health Insider. (2007). "DH to lift hospital mobile phone ban." http://www.e-health-insider.com/news/item.cfm? ID=2542.

[51] Chi-Kit, T., C. Kwok-Hung, et al. (2009). "Electromagnetic Interference Immunity Testing of Medical Equipment to Second- and Third-Generation Mobile Phones." IEEE Transactions on Electromagnetic Compatibility, 51(3): 659-664.

[52] Ardavan, M., K. Schmitt, et al. (2010). "A preliminary assessment of EMI control policies in hospitals." 14th International Symposium on Antenna Technology and Applied Electromagnetics and the American Electromagnetics Conference.

[53] Witters, D., S. Seidman, et al. (2010). "EMC and wireless healthcare." Asia-Pacific Symposium on Electromagnetic Compatibility.

[54] Phond Phunchongharn, D. N., Ekram Hossain and Sergio Camorlinga (2010). "An EMI-Aware Prioritized Wireless Access Scheme for e-Health Applications in Hospital Environments." IEEE transactions on information technology in biomedicine, 14(5): 1247-1258.

[55] Phunchongharn, P., E. Hossain, et al. (2010). "A cognitive radio system for e-health applications in a hospital environment." IEEE Wireless Communications, 17(1): 20-28.

[56] Phunchongharn, P., D. Niyato, et al. (2010). "An EMI-Aware Prioritized Wireless Access Scheme for e-Health Applications in Hospital Environments." IEEE Transactions on Information Technology in Biomedicine, 14(5): 1247-1258.

[57] Salvador, C. H., M. P. Carrasco, et al. (2005). "Airmed-cardio: a GSM and Internet services-based system for out-of-hospital follow-up of cardiac patients." IEEE Transactions on Information Technology in Biomedicine, 9(1): 73-85.

[58] Niyato, D., E. Hossain, et al. (2009). "Remote patient monitoring service using heterogeneous wireless access networks: architecture and optimization." IEEE Journal on Selected Areas in Communications, 27(4): 412-423.

[59] Ghevondian, N. and N. Hung (1997). "Using fuzzy logic reasoning for monitoring hypoglycaemia in diabetic patients." IEEE conference on engineering in Medicine and Biology Society.

[60] Medical electrical equipment, Part 1"C2 (2003): General Requirements for Safety, Collateral Standard: Electromagnetic Compatibility, Requirements and Test, National Standard of Canada CAN/CSA-C22.2 No. 60601-1-2:03 (Adopted IEC 60601-1-2:2001).

[61] Maaref, A. and S. Aissa (2005). "Closed-form expressions for the outage and ergodic Shannon capacity of MIMO MRC systems." IEEE Transactions on Communications 53(7): 1092-1095.

[62] Maaref, A. and S. Aissa (2005). "Spectral efficiency limitations of maximum ratio transmission in the presence of channel estimation errors." IEEE 62nd Vehicular Technology Conference.

In: Health Informatics
Editor: Naveen Chilamkurti

ISBN: 978-1-61942-265-0
© 2013 Nova Science Publishers, Inc.

Chapter 4

ARCHITECTURE AND PROTOCOLS FOR BODY SENSOR NETWORKS

Sudip Misra, Judhistir Mahapatro* and Amit Kumar Mandal**

School of Information Technology
Indian Institute of Technology
Kharagpur – West Bengal, India.

ABSTRACT

Recently there has been an upsurge of research interest on Body Sensor Networks (BSNs). In BSNs, biomedical sensor nodes are deployed in the different parts of the human physiological system. These nodes interconnect to form a network through which vital physiological information sensed by the sensors deployed on the human body are sent to the control center for further processing and patient monitoring. The expeditious advancements in biomedical sensors, low power integrated circuits, short range RF transceivers and low-cost antennas (directional/ omni-directional) have helped in the realization of BSNs. Increased network reliability, ease of accessibility, real-time monitoring of patients are fundamental research challenges of concern in BSNs. BSNs have

* smisra@sit.iitkgp.ernet.in
* judhistir.java@gmail.com
* amiit.mandal@gmail.com

specific characteristics that make them unique over regular Wireless Sensor Networks (WSNs). Unlike regular WSNs, mobility models for BSNs are influenced by the human body movement. The low transmitted power signal of the nodes in BSNs minimizes the risk of health hazards. By having implanted sensors closer to the suspected areas of the human body, it is possible to analyze the information about the chronological state of the different parts of the body through offline or online means, depending upon the severity of the disease affecting the body. For instance, data transaction would be in non-real-time for monitoring the metabolic rate of cells (chemical reaction), insulin/glucagon level in blood, blood pressure, heart-rate, lungs-rate, blood viscosity of an athletic, and can be analyzed using offline techniques. On the contrary, a group of cancerous cells have to be monitored in an online manner. In recent years, many protocols and algorithms have been proposed for BSNs. Some of the popular ones include medium access control (MAC) protocols (e.g., H-MAC and BSN-MAC) and Delay-Tolerant Network (DTN) —in this case Body-DTN— are mostly concerned. In this chapter we review the architecture and protocols for BSNs.

1. INTRODUCTION

The rapid technological growth in wearable bio-medical sensors, low power integrated circuits, short range RF transceivers, and low-cost antennas (directional or omni-directional) leads to shape the growth of BSNs. BSNs are different from other wireless network technologies due to their unique features such latency and data rate. But they provide interfaces to other wireless communication networks such as Wi-Fi, Wi-MAX, and WSN.

The physiological sensors may be either placed on the human body or may be implanted into the tissues of the body using incisive techniques. Unlike in the case of other WSN application domains, where it is assumed that the sensor nodes are non-removable, non-rechargeable and non-replaceable, in BSNs it is possible, and in fact, it is an important requirement for performing these operations, when the battery energy gets depleted or when a node becomes non-functional. However, it should not be construed from the above statements that energy-efficiency is not a matter of prime importance in BSNs. In fact, it is important that the protocols designed for BSNs should be energy-efficient, fault-tolerant, and reliable. Our findings show that there exists ample scope of research on these aspects of BNSs. As it goes by the saying, "prevention is better than cure", it is important to have regular/periodic monitoring of health of vital physiological parameters (e.g., blood pressure, glucose level, and pulse rate) of patients. Ordinarily, when a patient requires medical attention, he/she has to periodically travel to a hospital or clinic. The on-duty doctor or nurse periodically checks the observed symptoms, performs some tests, and finally prepares the diagnostic report. Some diseases such as cancer develop in tissues requiring early detection; otherwise, the disease may lead to fatality. Taking the example of cancer, studies have shown that the cancerous cells emit very small quantity of nitric oxide, which affects the blood present around the cancerous tumor. The sensor network technology can offer help in this case. It has been shown that early detection of cancer can be achieved through a sensor (with the ability to detect changes in blood) placed at the suspect locations of human body [1].

Currently, there are a number of research activities being undertaken worldwide focusing on investigating using the human body as a medium of communication – a mechanism termed as *body channel communication* (BCC) [2]. In BCC, the transmitting signals do not interfere with the signals of other Radio Frequency (RF) enabled external devices present in the vicinity. The characteristics of the body channel using a relation as a function of transmission distance, frequency, transmission power, and received power have been analyzed. In Ref. [2], the authors have analyzed that the body channel shows a characteristic akin to a band-pass with 120 MHz bandwidth, and the relation inferred would be useful in calculating the energy-efficient frequency range. Also, by graph analysis, the optimized frequency band for the body channel has been found to be 10-100 MHz in order to maximize the transmission distance of the sensor node. An energy-efficient networking protocol using body channel communication (BCC) has also been proposed in [2].

In recent years, many protocols and algorithms have been proposed for BSNs, but only a few of them are operational in practice. However, the impediments in the growth of this field are yet to be investigated. Many researchers, working in this field of research, have been working on various protocols at different levels of the protocol stack of BSNs.

BSNs can be used to sense and monitor continuously some activities and actions of human body such as metabolic rate of cells (chemical reaction), insulin/glucagon level in blood, blood pressure, heart-rate, lungs-rate, and blood viscosity. These autonomous sensors have ultra low transmission power and that they cannot directly send sensed information to an aggregator, which is connected to the Access Point (AP). The sensed information, which is encapsulated in the form of packets, should be routed through some intermediate nodes over the network to the aggregator. The selection of an optimized path over the BSN to route a data packet from the source node to the sink node could be based on some routing metrics. One such basic metric is the *hop count*.

In BSNs, the data sensed by the different sensors attached to various parts of a human body are sent hop-by-hop to an aggregator. As it appears, the help of intermediate nodes is extremely significant in relaying the data along the path over the network. It seems to be a static network because they are fixed on human body. As the communication progresses over time, the on-body sensor nodes becomes mobile due to high degree of dynamism of parts of the body. These autonomous sensors are used to sense the ambulatory functions of a human body spontaneously. The real-time data acquired in the process are sent over the BSN to the aggregator, and, if necessary, the data packets can be sent to a nearby hospital or clinic over the Internet through a wireless access point which is connected to the aggregator. It can be inferred from the above that for supporting such applications, highly reliable, stable, and fault-tolerant network protocols are required.

The rest of the chapter is organized as follows. In Section 2, we discuss the fundamental concepts behind WSN. In Section 3, we discuss the architecture of a typical BSN and the specific issues and features of BSN that make them unique. In Sections 4 and 5, we discuss some of the MAC and routing protocols for BSN. Finally, we summarize and conclude in Section 6.

2. WIRELESS SENSOR NETWORKS

A WSN consists of a large number of small-sized sensing devices (or sensors) widely deployed in a geographical area, where these devices are capable of sensing the physical phenomena in their surroundings. The nodes have limited computational power and resources. The main components of a sensor node include a transceiver, a processor, a memory unit, and a power unit. The sensors are battery-powered. They are always in any of the following three states: sensing, listening, and idle. More energy is consumed by the communication operation as compared to sensing and listening. As the sensor nodes are energy-constrained and have low transmission range, they cannot transmit the sensed data directly to the base station or sink which is strategically placed at some location in the region. The data sensed by a node in WSN can be sent hop-by-hop to the sink. In other words, a sensor node sends the data to one or more of its neighbors. Further, the neighbors relay the received data packets to their neighbors, and eventually the packet reaches the sink. The above process is also shown in Figure 1.

Figure 1 shows a network consisting of small-sized sensor nodes deployed in a geographical terrain. These sensor nodes have low-power, short distance transmission capability, and low data-rate components to meet the low-cost demand without sacrificing any of the basic requirements such as sensing and data relaying. Therefore, all the classical wireless protocols that operate at high data rate and are computationally intensive are not suitable for WSN. For example, IEEE 802.11b operates in the ISM band at 2.4 GHz with data rate of 11 Mbps, by which the aims at low expenditure for the infrastructure of WSN cannot be achieved. For example, we can use IEEE 802.11b, which operates in the ISM band at 2.4 GHz with data rate of 11 Mbps, but we need to have the sensor nodes equipped with more memory, power, and processing capability so as to see the desired performance of the IEEE 802.11b standard. This makes it challenging to design low-cost sensor nodes based on this standard. In order to address this, currently, the ZigBee (IEEE 802.15.4) [7, 8] standard is being explored for use in a wide range of WSN applications such as surveillance of agricultural field, health-care, military, and mining.

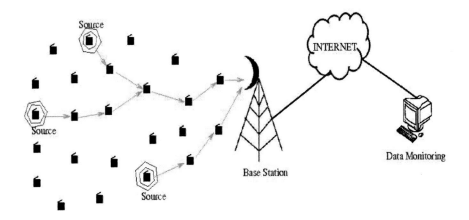

Figure 1. Wireless Sensor Network.

As we will see later in this section, a BSN is different from a WSN. But still it shares many common features with a WSN. Even many protocols that have been specifically proposed for WSN are not well suited for BSN.

The following features (adopted mostly from [3, 4]) distinguish a BSN from a WSN:

I.   **Density of Node:** The medical sensor nodes are placed according to their anatomical position on the human body, in order to measure specific physiological actions such as the lungs rate. For example, a sensor node that is placed for sensing the heart-rate of a human being should be placed over or near to the chest. The placement and replacement of sensor nodes in the appropriate locations on the human body are done manually and all the sensor nodes confined to the human body are accessible to the network operator. On contrary, the sensor nodes in WSN are strategically thrown into an area for the monitoring of different events, for example, monitoring of the habitats in a forest. In case of WSN, the failure of nodes is common and it is very hard in an actual sensor network deployment for the network operator to reach the faulty nodes. For this reason, they are densely deployed in order to increase the connectivity among them, so that the failure of some of sensor nodes does not affect the performance of WSNs [3].

II.   **Latency:** The improved reliability and energy consumption are the stringent requirements of any application of WSN. Additionally, there are different demands for the end-to-end delay by the users of the applications of WSNs, where the application involves transferring of real-time data from one end to the other within some specified time period. Apparently, the end-to-end delay is traded so as to get improved reliability and energy consumption in WSNs, whose sensor nodes are powered by the batteries. Therefore, it is necessary to have proper distribution of energy consumption among the sensor nodes in order to maximize the network life-time. Additionally, energy conservation at both the device and protocol levels is crucial because the replacement of batteries of sensor nodes is more difficult task than in BSN. Also, it seems that the reliability increases with respect to the increased battery life-time of sensor nodes in WSN. Hence, it is required to maximize the battery life-time of sensor nodes with higher end-to-end delay [3]. In case of BSN, the demand for the low end-to-end delay or latency from the medical applications may be considered and, of course, there is no need to maximize the battery life-time because of the ease of replacement of sensor nodes.

III.   **Security:** Compared to WSN, in BSN, stricter security mechanisms are required in order to provide privacy of health information of a patient [3].

IV.   **Low-Power Node:** Compared to WSN, in BSN, very low transmit-power enabled node is needed to avoid health concerns of an individual and channel interference [3].

V.   **Mobility:** The nodes in BSNs follow the same mobility pattern as the movement of limbs and other body parts, whereas the sensors in WSN are usually considered stationary (except in mobile sensor networks).

VI.   **Data-Rate Requirement:** The sensors such as EEG, ECG, and EMG run at the date rate of Kbps, and the aggregated data at particular sensor nodes in BSN predominantly increases. Thus, the data rate at particular sensor nodes should be in the order of few Kbps or even Mbps [4]. The events or physiological activities of the human body must be sensed periodically and the real-time data can be sent to an aggregator, but most WSN are event-driven, wherein the events occur at an irregular interval. So, BSN applications require a data stream with stable data rate as compared to WSN.

There may be more number of possible paths from the same source to the base station via intermediate relay nodes. However, one path should be selected in order to save the overall bandwidth and energy consumption. There has been tremendous research in developing and designing robust protocols for network layer and MAC layer. LEACH and PEGASIS are both examples of network layer protocol for WSN. S-MAC [5] and T-MAC [6] are both examples of the MAC layer protocol for WSN. Examples of BSN MAC protocols include H-MAC, B-MAC, and CICADA. These protocols are explained in Section 4.

3. INTERNET-BASED ARCHITECTURE OF BSN

In recent years, research on BSN has gained widespread attention, because of the attractive ability of these networks for automated healthcare monitoring. As discussed earlier, in typical BSN applications, the nodes in these networks are placed on the human beings in order to monitor the health conditions of patients in real-time, instead of on a regular check basis by booking an appointment in a clinic or a hospital.

In a BSN, the medium for communication used is wireless, instead of wired, thereby aiding in the portability of the network system. In addition, the movements of different organs of a human body would not affect the system. There are two types of wireless communication in BSN: (i) Body channel communication (BCC), and (ii) RF-radio communication. BCC has an advantage over RF communication in that there is no interference with other external RF devices when we use BCC. The human body is used as the channel for achieving seamless communication. On the other hand, it incurs more path loss when the two communicating devices are not in line-of-sight as one is placed on the anterior side of human body and the other placed on the posterior side of the human body.

Three types of bio-sensor installation methods are normally suggested for BSNs. They are *invasive*, *non-invasive* and *implanted* [16]. A non-invasive method is more common in BSNs than an invasive method, because of the obvious reasons of ease of installation externally on the body. Implanted sensors are placed using surgical techniques and they are supposed to be inside the body for more than a year. These sensors have also been classified based on the design that includes a resistor, capacitor, inductor or piezoelectric based sensing technology. Respectively, they are also named as *resistive*, *capacitive*, *inductive* and *piezoelectric sensor*. Unlike other sensors, a piezoelectric sensor is bidirectional. It can also work as an actuator which can convert the electrical signal received from the sensor into the physical action. The physiological sensors used for the health monitoring are given below:

I.   **EEG Sensor:** It is a small electrode that is attached to the scalp of the human head and is used to record the electrical activity across the scalp produced by the neurons within the brain. They can also forward the sensed data directly or via an intermediate node to an aggregator or a PDA which is named as HEAD (as shown in Figure 2).

II. **EMG Sensor:** It is intended to record the electrical signals that are generated by the muscles of human body when it undergoes expansion or contraction. The conduction of impulses carried by the nerves to the muscles from the brain is recorded using it.

III. **Motion Sensor:** A non-invasive motion sensor is often used to quantify the movement of an object by determining the change in its speed, but herein the object may be anything related to the body parts. Motion sensors are often required in applications such as sports, modeling, and health care. In addition, a motion sensor can be used for monitoring the gait and physical movement of a person. For example, a knee-sensor is useful in finding whether the person is running, walking or kneeling down.

IV. **Blood-Pressure Sensor:** The systolic and diastolic pressure of a person can be measured using the non-invasive blood pressure sensor. In other words, the systolic pressure is the pressure exerted on the wall of blood vessels by the blood flow when the heart is beating and the diastolic pressure is the pressure exerted on the wall of blood vessels when the heart is on resting position.

V. **Temperature Sensor:** Temperature generated inside the human body because of the chemical reaction in the cells can be recorded in real-time using a temperature sensor.

VI. **Glucose Sensor:** The concentration of glucose in the circulating blood of a human being can be measured using a non-invasive sensor that uses infrared light technique. The classical method of measuring the concentration of glucose in blood requires pricking on the tip of a finger and then smearing the blood on a glass strip. But regularly pricking on the same finger(s) can damage the finger tissue. For a diabetic patient it may be necessary to take out blood at least once a day from the body in order to monitor the glucose level. Blood glucose monitoring methods that use non-invasive sensors are more beneficial than the ones that use the classical ones.

VII. **Pressure Sensor:** The body/blood/enzymatic pressure exerted on the sensing mechanisms can be measured using the piezoelectric effect of quartz material of a piezoelectric sensor. For example, the pressure sensors in the footwears are used to monitor the pressure dissipation around the foot. It works similar to how the touch-screen application of an ATM machine works.

VIII. **ECG Sensor:** ECG is a mechanism which presents the heart's electrical activity on a screen or paper in the form of line graph. In case of a 12-lead ECG, six electrodes are placed around the chest, two electrodes are situated on limbs; one of them is placed on the right limb and other on the left limb and each of the remaining two are situated on right and left legs. Usually twelve different signals from twelve leads are recorded at the same time where a lead forms by pair of electrodes. Furthermore, the traced potential differences between these electrodes across all the leads are recorded using the ECG recorder for the later analysis of ECG of a human being. Of course, these ECG electrodes use non-invasive sensing technology.

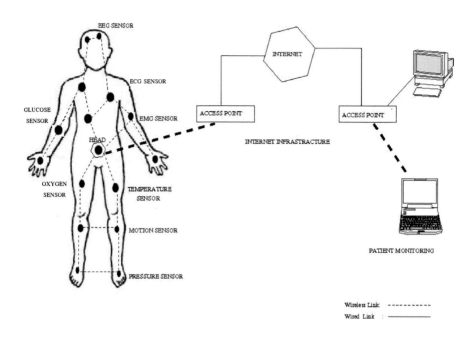

Figure 2. Internet-Based Architecture of BSN.

As sensors in BSN are powered by the battery, the medical application demands low-ultra power consumption at every node by its data-transfer and computation operations. Further, it is also required to have high data rate because of the requirement for transferring real-time data. So, it is required to have a compatible standard which supports very low power consumption and high data-rate required for medical applications. There has been existing standards, but they are suitable fully or partially depending on the type of requirement of an application. Although the Bluetooth standard consumes more power, it could be applicable for the health-care applications that require inter-BSN communications. BSN-to-BSN communication can be achieved using Bluetooth radio technology because of Bluetooth's support for maximum data-rate of 3 Mbps and operate in the 2.4 GHz ISM band. Fortunately, we have another standard that is Bluetooth low power technology which is expected to provide the data-rate up to 1 Mbps and it operates in the 2.4 GHz ISM band. But the devices run with this standard succumb to interference from all other ubiquitous devices running in the same ISM band.

As mentioned earlier, ZigBee/IEEE 802.15.4 [7, 8] is one of the existing standards, and it is best suited for intra-BSN communication, because of its low power consumption. But it can support data-rate up to 250 kbps. The data rate is 250 kbps with 16 channels between 2400 – 2483.5 MHz which is made available all over the world. This expected data-rate is not sufficient for BSN, where high data streaming is required. The video streaming applications based on X-rays or ultrasounds need high data-rate. The ZigBee standard supported radio devices can be divided into two types — the Full Function Device (FFD) and Reduced Function Device (RFD). In contrast to the RFD, its data rate is more and also it can act as coordinator in the network. Furthermore, it can communicate with RFDs and other FFDs in the network, but a RFD can only communicate to a FFD.

ZigBee [7] has the support for three different network topologies: *star*, *mesh*, and *cluster tree*. In a star topology, each candidate node in the network communicates with the coordinator which is a FFD. The purpose of the coordinator is to control and manage the network. Therefore, at least one FFD must exist in order to become the coordinator. The star topology is simpler amongst all the three topologies and also the corresponding routing protocols are relatively light-weight. In a mesh topology, any node can communicate directly with any other node. Sometime it can also communicate between any two nodes using multi-hop. The direct communication between any two nodes is possible only when they are in range of one another. The mesh topology also has a coordinator. It is also more resilient to path failures because it uses a multi-path approach. Thus, it ensures high reliability of data delivery to the controller or a coordinator.

A cluster tree topology consists of a tree of clusters with a personal area network (PAN) coordinator (a coordinator for overall tree). A cluster is formed by a group of sensor nodes with a coordinator. In cluster tree topology, each sensor node should communicate with the coordinator of a cluster in order to communicate with all other sensor nodes over the network. This may be visualized and obtained by connecting the coordinator of two or more star topologies together, while each star topology is being treated as the cluster with a coordinator. The number of FFDs is more in cluster tree topology compared to that in the other topologies mentioned above. One of the coordinators in the network is a PAN coordinator and it is also called as a controller.

We need to pass the gathered data of HEAD instantly over an Internet-Based infrastructure to a nearby hospital or a doctor who sits with a computer in office away from the hospital ward, as shown in Figure 2. The HEAD device or the controller of the BSN talks to an AP which is in the vicinity of

BSN. The HEAD may use multiple-radio interface to communicate with the AP, as well as with the intra-BSN nodes.

4. MAC PROTOCOLS FOR BSN

The interfering nodes of shared medium of MAC pose two very serious problems in any wireless networks: (i) *Hidden terminal*, and (ii) *Exposed terminal*. The hidden terminal problem arises when two networked sensor nodes transmit at the same time to the same destination that leads to collision of data packets at the receiving node, which is present in between them as an intermediate node. This collision is seen because both the transmitting sensor nodes are not aware of each other as they are out of range of each other. The exposed terminal problem arises when one of the sensor nodes is not allowed to transmit its data because of its neighboring transmissions. For example, four sensor nodes A, B, C and D are placed on a line respectively where B is in the range of A and C, as well as C is in the range of B and D. Currently, B sends to A and at the same time C wants to send packets to D, but C is not allowed to transmit because C is in the range of B. Nonetheless, if C is allowed to send packets to D that does not lead to any collision because D is not in range of other two sensor nodes except C. The impact of the aforesaid problems can be partly reduced using handshaking messages RTS (Request to Send), CTS (Clear to Send), as well as directional antenna [17, 18].

The wireless network MAC protocols are broadly classified into either of the two major categories: contention-based or schedule-based. CSMA/CA and TDMA are the examples of contention-based and schedule-based respectively. In contention-based, the nodes contend for the same channel (medium), but the one who wins the competition will be assigned the medium. In scheduled-based, nodes are free from idle listening, control and packet collisions due to lack of competitors for the medium. Furthermore, the nodes are allowed to send their available traffic in the channel only during the assigned time-slot, but it needs strong clock synchronization techniques to provide tight synchronization among nodes. There are some well-known MAC protocols for WSNs such as S-MAC [5] and T-MAC [6]. S-MAC lets the nodes go for periodic sleep thereby reducing the listening time and the overall duty cycle. T-MAC improves the energy consumption over S-MAC using the duty cycle adaptively with respect to the adaptive traffic. Although BSN and WSN share some common characteristics, improved MAC protocols should be designed specifically for use in BSN. The MAC protocols that have been proposed for BSN are discussed below:

4.1. H-MAC

H-MAC [9] is a schedule-based MAC protocol for BSN, and it is specially designed for the star topology. In general, the designated coordinator in the star topology assigns a contention-free time-slot to the nodes and it also uses the periodic beacons to synchronize them. The coordinator of H-MAC uses the heartbeat rhythm information instead periodic beacon to synchronize all the sensor nodes in BSN. The network is relieved from the beacon signals and it achieves more energy conservation than in beacon-based TDMA thus prolonged the life-time of BSN.

4.2. BSN-MAC

BSN-MAC [10] is a BSN MAC protocol that is compatible with the IEEE 802.15.4 [8] standard, which provides 16 channels in the ISM band at 2.4GHz and it supports both the star and the peer-to-peer topologies. BSN-MAC is a low-ultra-power MAC developed specially for the star topology of a BSN. It classifies all the sensor nodes in a BSN into four types as follows: *constrained, unconstrained, highly constrained,* and *extremely constrained.* It is difficult to recharge batteries in the implanted sensor nodes in BSN applications. Therefore, they are extremely energy *constrained.* However, it is assumed that the coordinator or HEAD of a BSN is energy *unconstrained* and we can replace its battery. Depending on the applications it prioritizes the sensor nodes based on their criticality of energy for accessing the medium so as to improve the power consumption at the energy-critical sensor nodes. Also, BSN-MAC adaptively adjusts the parameters of the MAC protocol by exploiting the feedback information such as the current energy level from the sensors in the network.

4.3. CICADA

CICADA (Cascading Information retrieval by Controlling Access with Distributed Slot Assignment) [11] is a cross-layer BSN protocol. It uses the same packet for both medium access as well as routing. The protocol sets up a spanning tree, all the sensor nodes on the tree can only send the data up the tree to the sink, which is the root of the tree. This scheme is used to achieve collision-free transmission. In the beginning of each scheduling cycle, the tree assigns the time slots to all the sensor nodes. The protocol then divides this cycle into control sub-cycle and data sub-cycle. The control information is sent downward the tree during the control sub-cycle and during the data sub-cycle the sensed data are sent up the tree to the sink.

4.4. Other MAC Protocols

In addition to the protocols discussed in Sections 4.1-4.3, research works on improvising the reliability, energy efficiency, and end-to-end delay have been undertaken. In Ref. [19], the authors proposed a novel MAC protocol for the Wireless Body Area Networks (WBAN). This is specifically developed for the point-to-multipoint deployment of nodes. A cluster is formed from a set of slave nodes and a master node, where all the slave nodes want to join the cluster. The master in the cluster controls all the slave nodes to make seamless communication between the master and the slaves in order to avoid collision. The protocol undergoes three communication processes: *link establishment, wake-up service,* and *alarm.*

Link-establishment: The master sends a beacon on an available link. The slave node listens to the occupied channel to receive the beacon and sends back an acknowledgement when it gets the beacon. The master sends the sleep time and configuration data after it received the acknowledgement from the slave. One more time, they exchange the acknowledgment messages between them. Both nodes (master and slave) go to the sleep mode.

Wake-up: The slave and master wake up at the same time, but the master sends a specialized beacon expecting for the recent data from the slaves. The slaves then send their data in the previously assigned slots. The master provides new sleep time after receiving the acknowledgement from the slaves. Thereafter, the slave and master go to the sleep mode.

Alarm: When a slave wants to send its data without waiting for the next wake-up, and if it is enabled then the master sends message to all the slaves sequentially. A back-off algorithm is used to avoid idle listening of nodes.

In [20], the authors proposed an energy-efficient MAC for Patient Personal Area Networks (PPAN). It consists of a master and many slaves. The master node administrates the communication between the master and slaves to achieve the better performance in terms of energy consumption. There are two reasons behind the increased energy consumption of nodes: collision and overhearing. They are common in sensor networks because their transmission range intersects. In the protocol, the communication time is divided into four slots and they are Transmit (Tx), Receive (Rx), Receive to Synchronize (Rsx), and Stand By Mode (Sb). The protocol is designed in such a way that the master and the slaves go to the standby mode at same time after the communication operations. The alteration of time slot has been used in order to avoid long run delay in the system. It uses optional acknowledge to reduce the unnecessary retransmission by piggy backing on to the ongoing data packets. On an unavailability of ongoing data packet, it can use an acknowledgement-type control packet for the purpose. This protocol becomes energy efficient by avoiding the overhearing, the collision and the retransmissions.

5. ROUTING PROTOCOLS FOR BSN

There is plethora of routing protocols for WSNs. They are not suitable for the BSN because the routing requirements by the applications of a BSN are different. The routing protocols that have been designed specifically for BSNs are summarized below:

5.1. BSDTN

The BSN routing protocols can be classified to belong to any of the two following data-transfer categories: real-time, and non-real-time. The applications such as monitoring of patient would require real-time packet routing where data packets are sent through intermediate nodes to the sink, which in turn relay the data packets to the beyond-on-body server or AP which is connected to Internet. The application that the monitoring of athlete's actions would not require real-time data transfer as the collected data could be required at later point of time for the analysis purpose. The high degree of posture changes of a human being and the short RF range could cause often network partitions or disconnections in BSN topologies, in resulting Body Sensor Delay Tolerant Network (BSDTN). The frequent topological partitioning may not be supported in case of the real-time traffic based applications like patient monitoring, but the network partitioning may be supported in the case of non-real-time traffic applications like an athlete's physiology monitoring using the on-body DTN packet routing across the disconnected partitions. In Ref. [12], the proposed Body Sensor DTN routing protocol is working on the probabilistic framework for likelihood of a link to be connected between two sensor nodes during a discrete time slot.

5.2. Temperature Aware Routing Protocols

One application of a BSN seeks to implant the sensor nodes in human bodies and these implanted sensor nodes to be used for monitoring the glucose level, the oxygen level, and detecting of cancer. The implanted sensor nodes transmit the sensed data to the end terminals, such as PDAs, using the wireless connectivity. In general, the communication between the implanted sensors and the terminals often use multi-hop transmissions to improve the energy consumption. As long as the implanted sensor nodes involve in the transmission and processing the generating temperature of these sensors rises. However, the temperature that is generated by the overheated sensor nodes may cause damage to the surrounding tissues. It is necessary that the tissues should be given extreme care because they are very delicate. The implanted sensor nodes are supposed to be there inside the human bodies for the long term monitoring, and due to the long term monitoring the temperature of sensor nodes rises up. Thus, the routing protocols need to be designed to suppress the increasing temperature of the implanted nodes in the network. Four thermal aware routing protocols were proposed and they are thermal-aware routing algorithm (TARA) [13], least temperature routing (LTR) protocol [14], adaptive least temperature routing (ALTR) [14] protocol, and least total-route-temperature (LTRT) [15] protocol. In this section, we introduce these four temperature aware routing protocols.

5.2.1. TARA

The routing protocol Thermal Aware Routing Algorithm (TARA) [13], is designed to provide the temperature aware routing capability to the implanted sensor nodes in BSNs. Initially, every node in the network exchanges the localized temperature information with their neighbors to know the list of neighbors, as well as to know that how many hops they are away from the others. The sensor node detects the hot spots around it before it sends the data to the destination over the route. In TARA, the hot spot is defined as the areas that have the sensor nodes with increased temperature that is more than the predefined threshold temperature limit. A sender sends a packet that is destined for the destination to a neighbor which is on the way to the destination and not a hot spot, and so on. If the current sensor node detects the neighbors (except the sender) as the hot spots then it sends back the received packet to the sender again, and the sender selects an alternative node to the destination, and if the sender does not find an alternative node to send the packet to the destination then it sends back to its previous node, and so on. When those sensor nodes cooled down to low temperature that is less than the predefined threshold limit of temperature, and it again includes them as the new sensor nodes in its routing. This mechanism can work effectively when every sensor nodes in a BSN must know the current temperature level of their neighbors. The generation of temperature of a sensor node is due the transmission radiation. Therefore, every sensor node in the network always by listening to their neighbor's packets to know the temperature changes in their neighbors.

5.2.2. LTR

The routing protocol, Least Temperature Routing (LTR) protocol [14], is also designed to avoid the hot spot while building a route so as to reduce the temperature at a particular implanted sensor node. Every sensor node in the BSN is maintaining the updated record of their neighbor's temperature as it is explained in TARA. Unlike TARA, LTR selects a neighbor having the least temperature or the coolest neighbor which will be the next node to receive and forward the data packets, if the selected neighbor is the destination of the packet then it can directly send the packets. The packet includes a basic routing metric that is MAX_HOPCOUNT to limit it to a certain number of hops aiming to improvise utilization of bandwidth. When a sensor node receives a packet, it compares the hop-count of the packet with the predefined MAX_HOPCOUNT. If the hop-count exceeds the predefined MAX_ HOPCOUNT, it will throw the packet away from the network. Also, it maintains a table to record the list of nodes that just passed the packets to avoid the loop transmission that is the packet sent by the sender comes back.

5.2.3. ALTR

The adaptive least temperature routing (ALTR) protocol [14] is designed to minimize the packet delivery delay by extending the LTR protocol. In ALTR, when a sensor node has a packet to forward it checks whether the hop-count of the packet is less than or equal to the predefined MAX_ HOP COUNT_ADAPTIVE. On successful, the node forwards the packet using LTR protocol. Otherwise, use the shortest hop routing (SHR) algorithm to send the packet to the destination.

5.2.4. LTRT

In TARA, LTR and ALTR, the sensor nodes always choose the coolest neighbor to forward the packets, but it does not check whether the coolest neighbor is in towards the destination. However, the total number of hops and total temperature on the route to the destination is increased.

The least total-route-temperature (LTRT) protocol [15] is designed to minimize the bandwidth that is consumed due to the longer stay of packets over the network. In this protocol, it applies the single-source shortest path problem algorithms (e.g., Dijkstra's algorithm) of graph theory after transforming the BSN into a graph, where each sensor node is represented as a vertex and an edge between the sensor node and its direct neighbor. The weight value of the link (edge) between the node and its neighbor is the generated temperature of the neighbor. For example, an edge from a sensor node 'A' to a neighbor 'B' is assigned with a weight (the temperature of the sensor node 'A'). It selects the routes with least total from a sender or source to the destination, so the number of hops on a route is reduced. Therefore, it minimizes the consumption of bandwidth, as well as the packet delivery delay. On the other hand, one tradeoff of this protocol is that it needs the temperature of all sensors to be exchanged among them, which increases the temperature of the network.

5.3. Other Routing Protocols

A mobile wireless body area sensor network (MWBASN) consists of sensor nodes deployed on human beings when they move these nodes self-configured to form a network. In MWBASN, each wearable sensor node employs a GPS (Global Positioning System) to know its global geographical position. Each node can calculate the distance between itself and the sink node. The authors in the paper [21] proposed an efficient location-based routing protocol for MWBASN. One of the neighbor nodes with maximum residual energy and minimum distance to the sink will be selected as a forwarding node.

In Ref. [22] the authors proposed a fuzzy-based AODV routing protocol for physiological monitoring using sensor networks. The protocol takes two fuzzy inputs such as RSSI (Received signal strength Indicator), and remaining energy of the nodes. The fuzzy inference approach was used to find out the optimized path over the network.

The frequent topology partitioning and continuous change of posture of a human body are common. In this paper [23], proposed a store and forward packet routing algorithm for BSNs.

6. SUMMARY AND CONCLUSIONS

The potential deployment of sensor nodes on a patient's body will be useful in providing the different physiological data at the same time and are made available to the nearby hospital on a real-time basis. In this Chapter, we discussed an Internet-Based architecture of BSN that has the wireless communication between the sensor nodes and between the HEAD node and the AP. We review some features of BSN that they distinguish it from WSNs. Also, we include different physiological sensors that are viable to sense the changes in the organs, the tissues and the cells of the body. The manufacturing companies of wearable biomedical sensors are rigorously trying to produce the sensor node of low power and smaller in size. Besides, it is required that a better MAC protocol in terms of energy saving. We review some of the MAC protocols in our chapter. The high degree of dynamism of a human body leads to the often partition of the network in BSN. The high reliable transmission of physiological data is required, as well as a routing protocol that should guarantee the delivery of packets to the destination. Also, the protocol should consume very less power for its routing. The continuous transmissions by a node that will increase its temperature and would damage the surrounding tissues. We discuss the techniques that they provide care while route the data without affecting the tissues or the organs of the body. We discussed the existing routing protocols for the BSN in this chapter. In the chapter, we intent to cover the recent advancements and researches towards the area of BSN.

ACKNOWLEDGMENTS

This work was partially supported by Council of Scientific and Industrial Research (CSIR), India, Grant Ref. No. 22(0419)/06/EMR-II.

REFERENCES

[1]   P. Neves, M. Stachyra, and J. Rodrigues, "Application of Wireless Sensor Networks to Healthcare Promotion," *Journal of Communications Software and Systems,* Vol. 4, No. 3, Dec. 2008, pp. 181-190.

[2]   J. Yoo, N. Cho, and H.J. Yoo, "Analysis of Body Sensor Network Using Human Body as the Channel," in *Proc. of the ICST International Conference on Body Area Networks* (BodyNets '08), Tempe, Arizona, USA, 2008.

[3]   M. Chen, S. Gonzalez, A. Vasilakos, H. Cao, and V. C. M. Leung, "Body Area Networks: A Survey," *Springer Mobile Network Applications,* # DOI 10.1007/s11036-010-0260-8, 2010.

[4]   B. Latre, B. Braem, I. Moerman, C. Blondia, and P. Demeester, "A Survey on Wireless Body Area Networks," www.pats.ua.ac.be/content/publications/2010/bbraem10wbansurvey.pdf , Accessed in Dec. 2010.

[5]   W. Ye, J. Heidemann, and D. Estrin, "An Energy-Efficient MAC Protocol for Wireless Sensor Networks," in *Proc. of 21st Annual Joint Conference of the IEEE Computer and Comm. Societies* (INFOCOM 2002), Vol. 3, 2002, pp. 1567-1576.

[6]   T. V. Dam, and K. Langendoen, "An adaptive energy-efficient MAC Protocol for Wireless Sensor Networks," in *Proc. of 1st ACM Conf. Embedded Networked Sensor Systems* (SenSys), Nov. 2003, pp. 171-180.

[7]   Zigbee Alliance, official web page: http://www.zigbee.org.

[8]   IEEE 802.15.4-2006, available:

[9]   http://standards.ieee.org/getieee802/download/802.15.4-200 6.pdf.

[10] H. Li, and J. Tan, "Heartbeat-Driven Medium-Access Control for Body Sensor Networks," *IEEE Transactions on Information Technology in Biomedicine,* Vol. 14, No. 1, Jan. 2010, pp. 44-51.

[11] H. Li, and J. Tan, "An Ultra-low-power Medium Access Control Protocol for Body Sensor Network," in *Proc. of 27th Annual International Conference of the Engineering in Medicine and Biology* (IEEE-EMBS 2005), China, Sept. 2005, pp. 2451-2454.

[12] B. Latre, B. Braem, I. Moerman, C. Blondia, and E. Reusens, "A Low-delay Protocols for Multihop Wireless Body Area Networks," in *Proc. of 4th Annual International Conference on Mobile and Ubiquitous Systems: Networking and Services* (MobiQuitous '07), 2007.

[13] M. Quwaider, and S. Biswas, "DTN Routing in Body Sensor Networks with Dynamic Postural Partitioning," *Elsevier Ad Hoc Networks 8 (2010)*, pp. 824-841.

[14] Q. Tang, N. Tummala, S.K.S. Gupta, and L. Schwiebert, "TARA: Thermal aware Routing Algorithm for Implanted Sensor Networks," in *Proc. of 1st IEEE International Conference on Distributed Computing in Sensor Systems* (DCOSS' 05), 2005, pp. 206-217.

[15] Bag, and M. A. Bassiouni, "Energy Efficient Thermal aware Routing Algorithms for Embedded Biomedical Sensor Networks," in Proc. of 1st IEEE International Workshop on Intelligent Systems Techniques for Wireless Sensor Network in Conjunction with the 3rd IEEE International Conference on Mobile Ad-hoc and Sensor Systems, Vancouver, BC, Canada, pp. 604–609.

[16] D. Takahashi, Y. Xiao, F. Hu, J. Chen, and Y. Sun, "Temperature-Aware Routing for Telemedicine Applications in Embedded Biomedical Sensor Networks," *Journal on Wireless Communications and Networking,* Article ID 572636, pp. 1-11.

[17] R.A. Peura and J.G. Webster, "Basic sensors and principles," in *Medical Instrumentation,* 4th ed., J.G. Webster, Ed. USA: John Wiley & Sons, Inc, pp. 45–90, 2010.

[18] Y. Takatsuka, K. Nagashima, M. Takata, M. Bandai, and T. Watanabe, "A Directional MAC Protocol for Practical Smart Antennas," in *Proc. of IEEE Global Telecommunications Conference*, Dec. 2006, pp. 1-6.

[19] P. Karn, "MACA - A New Channel Access Method for Packet Radio," in *Proc. of Amateur Radio 9th Computer Networking Conference*, Sept. 1990, pp. 134–140.

[20] O. Omeni, A. C. W. Wong, A. J. Burdett, C. Toumazou, "Energy Efficient Medium Access Protocol for Wireless Medical Body Area Sensor Networks," *IEEE Transactions on Biomedical Circuits and Systems*, Vol. 2, No. 4, Dec. 2008, pp. 251-259.

[21] E. Lamprinos, A. Prentza, E. Sakka, and D. Koutsouris, "Energy-efficient MAC Protocol for Patient Personal Area Networks," in *Proc. of IEEE Engineering in Medicine and Biology 27th Annual Conference,* Shanghai, China, Sept. 2005, pp. 1-4.

[22] Kim, J. Kim, I. Lee, H. Lee, M. Yoon, and K. Han, "An Efficient Routing Protocol based on Position Information in Mobile Wireless Body Area Sensor Networks," in *Proc. of 1st International Conference on Networks & Communications*, DOI: 10.1109/NetCoM.2009.36.

[23] S. Yang, and K. Song, "An Adaptive Routing Protocol for Health Monitoring with a Sensor Network and Mobile Robot," in *Proc. of 36th Annual Conference on IEEE Idustrial Electronics Society*, Nov. 2010, pp. 2187-2192.

[24] M. Quwaider, and S. Biswas, "On-body Packet Routing Algorithms for Body Sensor Networks," in *Proc. of 1st International Conference on Networks and Communications,* Dec. 2009, pp. 171-177.

In: Health Informatics
Editor: Naveen Chilamkurti

ISBN: 978-1-61942-265-0
© 2013 Nova Science Publishers, Inc.

Chapter 5

INFORMATION AND COMMUNICATION TECHNOLOGIES ENABLED ASSISTED LIVING: AN INTEGRATION OF RFID AND WEB SERVICE

Mehmet S. Unluturk and Kaan Kurtel

Izmir University of Economics,
Faculty of Engineering and Computer Sciences,
Department of Software Engineering, Balcova, Izmir, Turkey

ABSTRACT

Everybody touches the healthcare issues. However, people 65 years and over need more than everyone and three primary forces affect their live: 1) their population increase; 2) they need more healthcare support; and 3) their incomes decrease. Availability of their care in their own homes is imperative because of the economic reasons and their choices where to live. Recent advancement in the information and communication technology are creating a new types of services. For instance, wireless communications and electronics have enabled the development of low-cost sensor networks and they can be employed in smart homes, e-healthcare applications and assisted living services. These statements show that there is a great promise in wireless technology and utilizing it in assisted living might be very beneficial to the elderly people. In this chapter, we propose a software architecture called the Location Windows Service (LWS) which integrates the Radio Frequency Identification (RFID) technology and the web service to build an assisted living system for elderly people at home. This architecture monitors the location of elderly people without interfering in their daily activities. Location information messages that are generated as the elderly move from room to room indicate that the elderly person is fit and healthy and going about their normal life. The communication must be timely enough to follow elderly people as they move from room to room without missing a location. Unacknowledged publishing, subscription filtering and short location change messages are also included in this software model to reduce the network traffic in large homes.

1. INTRODUCTION

Three major trends take the assisted living concept to a new level (Figure 1) [1]. The first trend is the major changes happening in the demographic profiles. In the mid of 19th century, the old age was defined as a social category and called the people over 50 as having old age. Now, in the developed countries, age 60+ years is called the old age. Despite the retirement age varies from country to country, the current legal and governmental frameworks in the member of EU countries and US have defined the average early retirement age as around 60. The World Health Organization's report [2] shows that the number of people over 65 years throughout the most stable and prosperous countries in the world is increasing. On the other hand, the online demographics of e-consumers continue to broaden with the fastest growth among teens, and older people [3].

The second trend is the economic reasons that affect the assisted living services. Internet-based changes in business and social life structures reshaped the existing customer profile. These new customers are now more familiar with internet based technologies and rapidly using more and more on-line applications. They have enough knowledge to use information and communication technologies (ICT) in their daily life. Also, the regulatory and financial barriers in the healthcare industry push the services to more economical means. However, good quality of healthcare system is still very expensive. At the beginning of the 21st century, shortages of hospital beds and medical people, limited budged options from government and private sector, as well as a decreased ratio of tax-paying workers are appearing as a reality. Moreover, people are always in need of better healthcare services and at the same time, their incomes are getting less as they get older. However, they still expect high standards with limited resources in hand from healthcare services. These dynamics change the role of hospitals in the health system and create the new type of healthcare systems such as telemedicine, smart home suppliers, and homecare organizations.

Finally, the third trend is the technology-based products and applications that offer new type of services. Medical device innovations, nurse call systems, smart home systems, *24x7 and real-time* remote monitoring systems are developed as better solutions for elderly people. Furthermore, these types of service ideas encourage more economic solutions and produce positive outcomes.

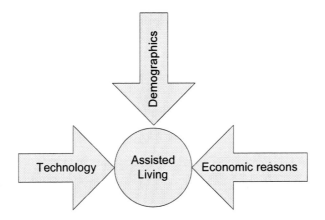

Figure 1. The assisted living services are affected by the three major trends.

Also, the several research studies [4-5] explored what a quality home care service should look like according to the elderly people:

- Need safety and better healthcare services
- Require good, safe transport and better healthcare services
- Need independence
- Live in their own homes
- Need good neighbors and friendly hearts
- See culturally specific languages, foods and activities
- Aids and adaptations
- Access to each area of the city
- Need information from health services

These results show that the most of the elderly people feel happy in their own homes. As the universal theme, "there is no place like home" that is mentioned in L. Frank Baum's book of *The Wonderful Wizard of Oz* is the best identifying words for their emotions.

Demographic realities, economic benefits of implemented e-Health solutions and technological challenges have been recently reviewed in the developed and developing countries. For instance, European Commission (EC) sets out a number of developing actions to improve the health-live balance for the elderly people. The Commission recognizes the power of ICTs to support the elderly people and estimated the smart homes market that is expected to triple between 2005 and 2020 [6]. The United States Department of Health & Human Services creates policies in all states and identified the assisted living services. The department reported several factors for the rapidly expanding assisted living industry; aging of the population, the preferences of the elderly people for settings other than nursing homes, the availability of private financing for development and construction of assisted living facilities, and public policies aimed at containing use of more nursing homes [7]. Such as, Australian Government, Department of Health and Ageing [8] produce programs and services of interest to the elderly people. The department reports that the number of the elderly people aged 65 years or more in Australia was estimated to be 2.6 million or around 13% of the total population. The proportion of older people in the population is projected to increase over time to 26% in 2051 and to 27% in 2101[9]. Additionally, the population of 65+ citizens is about 5,380,000 and it is 7.2% of general population in 2010 [10] in Turkey. In spite of the 12-18% in some developed EU member countries, the percentage of older people population is still low in Turkey. However, the increasing population of Turkey presents a barrier in the future. For that reason, the Turkish Ministry of Health develops some health programs in order to join the EU program too.

In this chapter, we would like to provide a software solution where we track the elderly people as they move from room to room indicate that the elderly person is fit and healthy and going about their normal life.

2. INFORMATION AND COMMUNICATION TECHNOLOGIES IN HEALTHCARE

Developing and sustaining a healthcare system with high quality care and outcomes have become more complex and more costly. The intersections of information and communication technologies help developers design better and less complex services and steer new ways in Health Informatics and Electronic Healthcare Applications. Because of the ability to support *the extreme bandwidth* demands in networks, the emergence and development of the internet and internet-based applications, and innovative internet computing systems, we can:

- speed up the healthcare applications;
- open up new possibilities in a number of health services;
- increase profitability and challenge economic prosperity;
- integrate healthcare system to healthcare supplies;
- link to medical practitioners and patients;
- provide more precise decision making ability;
- produce 24x7 and real-time remote monitoring;
- improve business fault tolerance, fault avoidance and alert managers to undesirable effects for the protection of life and high-quality healthcare services.

Some of the major application areas of ICT in healthcare are Hospital Information Systems (HIS), Nurse Call Systems, and Homecare Systems.

A HIS, also called Hospital Information Systems is a computer based system that is used to collect, store, quantify, and distribute clinical information and it provides patient specific operational aspects in the healthcare. The roles and goals of a HIS are; 1) enabling seamless and reliable to patient care, 2) increasing operational productivity, 3) enhancing decision making, and 4) improving collaboration and cooperation between medical staffs and patients.

These four points provide better alternative health care programs and plans for patients and elderlies, and also save their lives. For instance, pocket pagers, wireless interfaces, IR (Infrared) technologies and ADT (Admit, Discharge, Transfer) systems are all integrated into the nurse call systems to provide instant communication between a patient and a nurse. Furthermore, a nurse call system is an electrically functioned system by which patients can call from a bedside station or from a duty station. An intermittent tone is heard and a corridor lamp located outside the room starts blinking with a slower or a faster rate depending on the call origination. If a call originated from a bedside station is denoted by a slow intermittent tone and blinking rate. If the call is from a bathroom station, the intermittent tone blinking is more rapid. If a bedside call cord is pulled out, the tone and light operates at an even faster rate. The communication must be timely enough to follow staff, patient or equipment as they move from room to room, without missing a location. These communication devices are not a replacement for communicating with a patient face-to-face. Instead, they can enhance nurses' inherent communication with patients, reduce response time and improve the quality of care. With the help of IR technologies, nurses and equipment can be tracked within the hospital. The ADT system enables patient names to be displayed on nurses' pocket pagers or wireless phones. Furthermore, a software protocol can design for these devices to communicate with each other over the LAN (Local Area Network) to transmit nurse calls to pocket pagers and wireless phones carried by nurses. In the other side, a radio-frequency identifier (RFID) technology, web services and nurse call systems to establish, maintain, and monitor the location information of staff, patients, and equipment, so that this information can be displayed within the nurse call-based applications. This system is an integrated information system designed to manage the clinical aspects of a hospital.

The issue of these ICT with GSM based appliances is to provide guidance and oversight which helps us achieve extremely favorable results for the elderly and the disabled people.

3. ASSISTED LIVING SERVICES AND ICT

The Assisted Living Federation of America defines the assisted living as a long-term care option that combines housing, support services and healthcare, as needed [11]. The assisted living support services coordinate typically daily activities such as meals, medication, bathing, dressing and transportation and offer the following benefits to health organizations, elderly people and disables:

- Reduce medical costs and complexity of services
- Improve patient safety and quality of care
- Provide timely decision making
- Give the elderly people a choice of where to live

These benefits realize the real requirements of treating patients with medical chronic conditions, disabled with physical or mental disabilities, blind or deaf people, or people who are old enough so that they need some remote medical helps. Beyond these primary stakeholders, there are also other secondary stakeholders that include governments, hospitals, and third party payers, including insurance funds as well. Their primary needs to give better health care services. ICT is currently being employed in one of the surest ways to design and implement the new kind of support services in order to expand and realize these benefits.

The availability of communication and computer systems such as public switched telephone network, mobile communication network and the Internet can deliver cost-effective and convenient services for wireless sensors, workstations, mobile devices and RFID applications. They communicate with each other critic to interpret through their software implementations. All together, these devices can encapsulate in many medical applications and/or services. In this context, the assisted living services include a wide range of device examples, such as:

- **Communication devices**; pagers, cellular-phones, personal digital assistants (PDAs), radio frequency identification (RFIDs), tag locators.
- **Control devices**; sensors, bed-exit alarms, movement detectors, fire alarms.
- **Engineering devices**; manometers, speedometers, thermometers, pressure indicators and calorimeters which are the physical measurement instruments to measure the *physical entities.*

RFID is one of the brilliant technologies in the domain of ubiquitous assisted living services. Older people's activity inference is a core purpose to give better services. Putting RFID tags and sensors on the fine-grained activities of older people provide a wide understanding about their current situation, behavior and requests. The following six questions: When, Where, Who, What, How, and Why are critically important for these purposes [12]. ICT, RFID technologies and sensors provide service and process excellence throughout the home environment. They offer a fresh challenge to the stakeholders in the healthcare applications. For instance, finding misplaced items is one of the problems for elderly people and/or patients with medical chronic conditions such as dementia. Key rings, glasses, mobile phones and medicine organizer generally put in the wrong place and if they cannot quickly be found, the situation can be problematic. At this stage, items tagged by RFID tags and send some signals to the user interface, and then, user finds misplaced items easily. As another example, healthcare units must have some necessary information of the elderly people's daily and desired activities. Physical activities keep them both physically and mentally fit. For this, nurses want more control over elderly people when they live in their home environment. Moreover, nurses need to know what the latest situations of their patients are. Also, in case patients or elderly people fall down, immediate help should be provided. Motion detectors can produce some solutions for these problems. Patient's body, some daily objects such as refrigerator, toilet cover and television are the quite useful places to install the RFID tags and the motion detectors. If these devices do not generate any signals, because they are not used, then, this can be a problem indicator.

4. INTEGRATION

In this section, we proposed a location system that consists of badges, which are worn by elderly people or by their belongings (such as keys, watches, and glasses), a reader and a location windows service. Furthermore, we focus on reducing the communication traffic in the system.

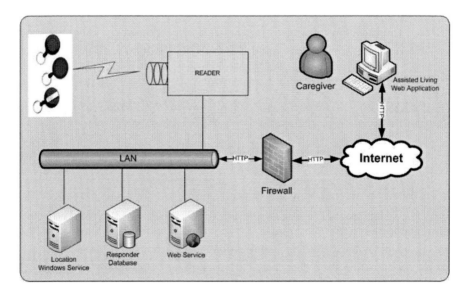

Figure 2. The architecture for the assisted living system that utilizes the RFID technology and the web service.

Figure 2 shows the basic architecture for the assisted living system. The antenna on the badge picks up the electro-magnetic energy beamed at it from a reader device and enables the badge to transmit its unique ID to the reader device, allowing the elderly person, or the owner to be, or the belonging to be remotely identified. The reader converts the radio waves coming back from the badge into digital information that can be transmitted to the location windows service for processing [13-17]. The location windows service writes these location data into the Responder database. The caregiver utilizes the assisted living web application that uses the web service to query the Responder database for real-time location data of the elderly people. The firewall is a defense scheme included in our system to prevent external intrusions.

Within the home-network, most of the messages are location change messages, and the communication traffic can be significant in large homes. Many assisted living systems that are integrated with sensor networks [18] do not consider any solutions for reducing the network traffic. These sensor networks generate an immense amount of information that creates additional overhead on network resources due to acknowledgments tracking and retransmission of missing location messages.

Overall system will have low reliability due to this high traffic. To reduce this traffic, we propose:

- *Unacknowledged Publishing*: The location change messages are published by the location windows service asynchronously to the assisted living web applications without acknowledgment. Message IDs inside the location change messages compensate for the lack of acknowledgement, enabling the assisted living web application to recognize a missed message and take appropriate action.
- *Subscription Filters*: Assisted living web applications request filters for their asynchronous badge movement messages. A filter string may contain one or more location types (Bath Room, Hallway, etc), or may contain one or more badge types (Elderly, Equipment, etc), with OR logic applied to all types within the filter string such as 'location type OR badge type'. In addition, both strings of filters can be simultaneously applied such as 'location type AND badge type'. The location windows service will deliver only the location messages that match the subscription filter. This will reduce the network traffic.
- *Short Location Messages*: Location changes, which comprise the majority of traffic, are passed as short messages containing the minimal information required to convey the change. Additional information is not required, but is allowed since it may reduce the overall system response time by eliminating the need for clients to look up information.

Our location/assisted living interface can be a unidirectional data-flow solution, with the assisted living accepting asynchronous badge movements from the location system without any acknowledgement returns (*Unacknowledged Publishing*). In addition, occasional assisted living queries for short location messages are provided to enhance the reliability of the interface. Either side in our design can also query for a list of location names, elderly names or equipment names. This minimizes any redundant configuration when a new hardware is added to our assisted living system. The next section talks about the location windows service.

4.1. Location Windows Service

The location windows service is designed to run unattended. It starts as soon as the operating system completes booting and runs even if no interactive user has logged in. The location windows service receives the location data change information from a reader (Figure 2), and generates the location change XML messages.

The windows service requires a database access to insert these location change XML messages into the Responder database for the web service. UML class diagram that is given in Figure 3 is implemented for the interface between the windows service and the database. Each database connection requires a connection object, and a command object. They are defined inside the interface called *IDatabaseAccess*. The main class *DatabaseAccess* holds a queue of connection objects. Connection objects are wrapped inside the *DBCon* class which implements the *IDatabaseAccess* interface. The windows service calls the main class *DatabaseAccess* to insert the location messages into the database. The *ExecuteNonQuery* method gets a connection object from the *Connection Queue* and a command object to write the location change XML messages into the database. The next section introduces the responder database.

4.2. Responder Database

The basic structure for the Responder database is to have the location change details defined inside the *ReceivedDateTime* and the *LocationMsgXML* database fields. The *LocationChange* object runs inside the location windows service. This object's purpose is to use the database access method that is illustrated in Section 4.1 to connect to the Responder database and insert the location change messages (Figure 4).

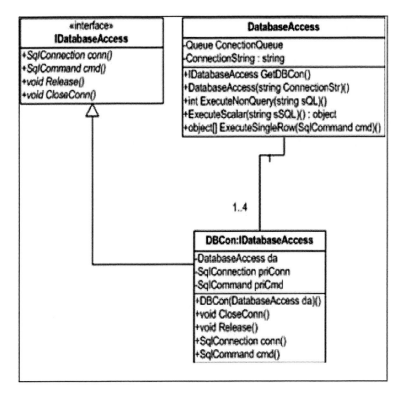

Figure 3. UML class diagram for the database access.

The web service uses the stored procedure that is given in Figure 5 to query the location change XML messages. Since the web service is stateless, we need to pull the responder database periodically. Information collected from the database is displayed on the web browser for the caregiver in the Section 4.4.

4.3. Web Service

The web service (Figure 2) is implemented as a .NET component that replies to HTTP requests from assisted living based applications that are formatted using the SOAP syntax [19]. Figure 6 shows the code sample for

GetLocationChanges web method. Assisted living clients use this method to query the *LocationChange* table inside the Responder database. The period for the query should be small enough so that assisted living based applications do not miss any locations. Also they do not want to process the same messages over and over again. To prevent that, clients provide the last message's date-time value processed by each client to the web method inside the *dt* argument.

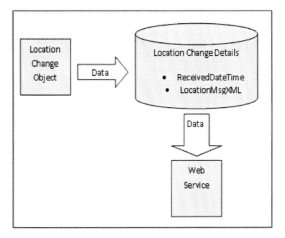

Figure 4. Structure of the Responder database.

The next section depicts an example for the assisted living based application and mentions the security.

4.4. Illustration of Assisted Living Based Application and Security

Figure 7 shows the display screen for the assisted living web application that uses the web service (Section 4.3) to query the Responder database. The assisted living based application processes each location change XML message and parses the details for Badge Number, Time Entered, Badge Type, Location, First Name, Last Name and MRNum (medical record number).

```
<LocationChg>
<MsgID>255</MsgID>
<BadgeID>104</BadgeID>
<LocName>bathroom</LocName>
```

```
<TimeEntered>11/23/2008 4:14:53 PM</TimeEntered>
<PrevLocName>hallway</PrevLocName>
<Elderly>
 <BadgeTypeName>grandfather</BadgeTypeName>
 <LastName>Doe</LastName>
 <FirstName>John</FirstName>
 <MiddleName>JD</MiddleName>
 <MRNum>7890</MRNum>
 </Elderly>
 </LocationChg>
```

```
PROCEDURE [dbo].[LocationChangeLoad]

        @dtmRecv datetime

AS

BEGIN

-- SET NOCOUNT ON added to prevent extra result sets
from

-- interfering with SELECT statements.

SET NOCOUNT ON;



-- Insert statements for procedure here

SELECT ReceivedDateTime, LocationMsgXML FROM
dbo.LocationChange

where ReceivedDateTime > @dtmRecv

ORDER BY ReceivedDateTime ASC

END
```

Figure 5. Sample stored procedure to query the location change XML messages.

```
[WebMethod] public DataSet GetLocationChanges(DateTime dt,

ref string sErr){

try

{ sErr="";

DataSet ds = new DataSet();

SqlConnection conn = new SqlConnection
        (System.Configuration.ConfigurationManager.AppSettings

["ConnectionString"]);

SqlCommand cmd = new SqlCommand("LocationChangeLoad", conn);

cmd.CommandType = CommandType.StoredProcedure;

SqlParameter param = new

SqlParameter("@dtmRecv",

SqlDbType.DateTime);

param.Value = dt;

cmd.Parameters.Add(param);

SqlDataAdapter da = new SqlDataAdapter(cmd);

da.Fill(ds); return ds;}

catch (Exception ex) { sErr=ex.ToString();  return null; }

}
```

Figure 6. Code sample for *GetLocationChanges* web method.

For example, the above XML message is received by the assisted living based application. It is parsed and the details for Badge Number, Time Entered, Badge Type, Location, First Name, Last Name and MRNum are written into the Responder database. The web application uses the web service to query the current locations of the elderly people and displays these details on the web application (Figure 7). John Doe whose badge number is 104 entered the bathroom on 11/23/2008 at 4:14:53 PM. This person's medical record number is 7890 that uniquely identifies him in assisted living system. His badge type tells us that the elderly person is a grandfather. Figure 7 also shows the current location information for Jane Doe. Jane Doe, grandmother, entered the hallway at 4:14:58 PM on 11/23/2008 whose badge number is 105 and medical record number is 7891. The current locations on the web application are refreshed automatically every two seconds or refreshed manually through the Refresh button by the care giver. Hence, the care giver can track the elderly person on any PC that has an internet connection using this web application.

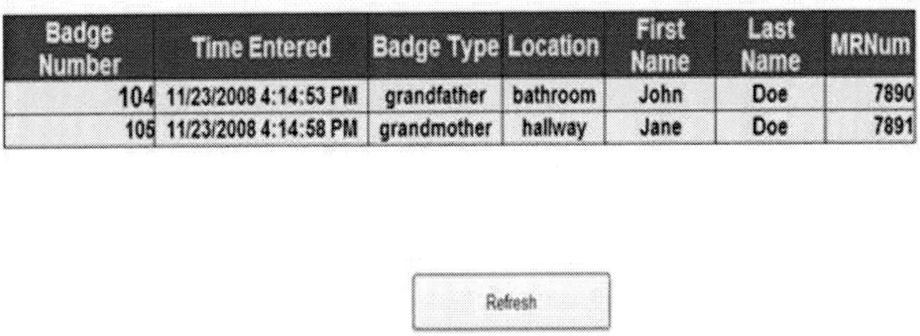

Badge Number	Time Entered	Badge Type	Location	First Name	Last Name	MRNum
104	11/23/2008 4:14:53 PM	grandfather	bathroom	John	Doe	7890
105	11/23/2008 4:14:58 PM	grandmother	hallway	Jane	Doe	7891

Refresh

Figure 7. An illustration of assisted living web application.

The use of the internet improves the communication between the elderly and the caregiver. Since the internet is a public environment, our proposed assisted living system can be invaded by hackers so that some defense schemes are needed. The objective of the defense schemes could be preventing illegal invasion, protecting the security of location messages, and providing the reliable assisted living system [20]. Illegal invasion can be divided into two forms. The first one is called a passive invasion whose purpose is to intercept the location messages and the second one is called an active invasion whose purpose is to modify the location message data in our assisted living system so that the system is unable to function normally. Currently, a firewall is applied to stop the external intrusions into the assisted living system (Figure 2). However, the location messages received by the assisted living web application are not encrypted. In this case, a vector network analyzer is adequate to intercept the non-encrypted location information. These location messages are confidential and need to be encrypted. Encrypting messages on the location windows service and decrypting on the assisted living web application take some time. Therefore, this process might bring some heavy burden to the overall system. The next section presents the conclusion.

5. CONCLUSION

This chapter develops a software architecture that leverages assisted living system using the RFID technology and the web service. This architecture can be also integrated into an existing nursing home where it has the ability to instantly locate the elderly person when he is in need. This can promote patient's safety and helps the care giver to provide better care. The care giver can decide the status of the room based on the location data. For example, either the room is available or it is in use. When the badge is placed in a discharge bin, this could be an indicator that the room needs to be cleaned and the housekeeping will be alerted. In our software architecture, the RFID data is read by the reader and is transmitted to the location windows service. The location windows service translates these into XML messages. The main database class inserts these messages into the database for the web service (Figure 2). The assisted living web application queries the database using the web service in a timely manner in order to follow elderly people as they move from room to room. Furthermore, using a central database in this software architecture minimizes the data entry. This architecture uses the unacknowledged publishing, the subscription filtering, and the short location change messages to reduce the network traffic. Each XML message is tagged with a message ID that can improve the overall reliability. Upon a recognized missed message ID, a client can query the location system for the missed location message. For future work, we would like to implement the assisted living web application on a mobile phone instead of on a PC. With the help of mobile phones, we can easily track our loved ones where ever we go and do not need to sit in front of a PC for that. These location messages are also confidential so that they need to be encrypted.

REFERENCES

[1]   Ambient Assisted Living Roadmap. (2010). *The European Ambient Assisted Living Innovation.* Ed. Ger van den Broek et al.

[2]   World Health Organization. Definition of an older or elderly person. 3 June 2011 <http://www.who.int/healthinfo/survey/ageingdefnolder/en/>.

[3]   Laudon K.C.; Traver C.G. E-commerce 2011; 7th edition; Pearson, 2011.

[4] Raynes N. et al. (2001). Getting older people's views on quality home care services. 3 June 2011 http://www.jrf.org.uk/publications/getting-older-peoples-views-quality-home-care-services

[5] Temple B; Glenister C; Raynes N. *Prioritising home care needs: research with older people from three ethnic minority community groups.* Institute for Health and Social Care Research, University of Salford, UK. 2002 May; 10(3):179-86.

[6] European Commission Information Society and Media. *Overview of the European strategy in ICT for Ageing Well.* October 2010.

[7] Catherine H.; Phillips C.D.; Rose M. 2000. *High Service or High Privacy Assisted Living Facilities, Their Residents and Staff: Results from a National Survey.* U.S. Department of Health and Human Services.

[8] Australian Government Department of Health and Ageing. 3 June 2011 <http://www.health.gov.au>.

[9] Australian Bureau of Statistics. 3 June 2011 <http://www.abs.gov.au>.

[10] Turkish Statistical Institute. 31 May 2011 <www.tuik.gov.tr>.

[11] Assisted Living Federation of America. 31 May 2011 <www.alfa.org>.

[12] Fishkin, K.P. "Ubiquitous computing challenges in recognizing and predicting human activity." *Proceedings of the International IEEE Conference on Fuzzy Systems,* Budapest, Hungary, 2004.

[13] Chowdhury B., and Khosla R. "RFID-based Hospital Real-time Patient Management System." *International Conference on Computer and Information Science.* 2007: 363-368.

[14] Canialosi A., Monaly J. E., and Yang S. C. "Leveraging RFID in Hospitals: Patient Life Cycle and Mobility Perspectives." *IEEE Applications & Practice,* September 2007: 18-23.

[15] Wu B., George R., and Shujaee K. "Architecting an Event-based Pervasive Sensing Environment in the Hospital." *3rd International IEEE Conference on Intelligent Systems,* 2006: 273-277.

[16] O'Halloran M., and Galvin M. "RFID Patient Tagging and Database System." *Int. Conf. On Mobile Comm. and Learn. Tech.* 2006: 162-167.

[17] Bravo J., Hervas R., Fuentes C., Chavira G., and Nava S. W. "Tagging for Nurse Care." *Pervasive Computing Technologies for Healthcare.* 2008: 305-307.

[18] Hongwei H., Youzhi X., Hairong Y., Saad M., and Hongke Z. "An Elderly Health Care System Using Wireless Sensor Networks At Home." *Third International Conference on Sensor Technology and Applications.* 2009:158-163.

[19]   Erl T. SOA: Principles of Service Design; Prentice Hall, 2008.
[20]   Chia-Hui L., Yu-Fang C., Tzer-Shyong C., and Sheng-De W. "The Enhancement of Security in Healthcare Information Systems." *Journal of Medical Systems*, DOI: 10.1007/s10916-010-9628-3.

In: Health Informatics
Editor: Naveen Chilamkurti

ISBN: 978-1-61942-265-0
© 2013 Nova Science Publishers, Inc.

Chapter 6

TOWARDS THE DESIGN OF TRULY PATIENT-CENTRED HEALTHCARE INFRASTRUCTURES: *A SOCIO-TECHNICAL APPROACH TO SELF-CARE*

Cristiano Storni and Liam J. Bannon**

Interaction Design Centre
Engineering and Research Building, University of Limerick
Limerick, Ireland

ABSTRACT

This paper examines a wide variety of issues concerning the doctor-patient relation, the medical model, the role of technology in self-care, and the issues of patient empowerment in current healthcare systems. The aim of the paper is to open up a debate concerning many of the background assumptions embedded in the rapidly expanding fields of self-care and home-health care, and to re-shape the role of technology in the design of a truly patient-centred healthcare system.

* Cristiano.storni@ul.ie
* liam.bannon@ul.ie; +353 61 202699

Keywords: socio-technical, practice, self-care, patient empowerment, biomedical model, infrastructure, patient-centred design.

PREAMBLE

This paper provides a perspective on the complex issues involved in designing and implementing open, flexible, participative, efficient and effective technical infrastructures and support systems in the healthcare field. The healthcare system is a very important part of the national infrastructure, affecting every citizen's quality of life. Debates rage over the most effective strategies and policies for delivering an effective service. New concepts within the sphere of civic participation in healthcare governance have raised serious questions as to the efficacy of the traditional medical model, with its reliance on institutionalization, high-tech solutions, and an expectation of patient compliance in the face of expert opinion. New models of care that explore more flexible strategies, such as home care and self-care regimens, and that recognize more fully the patient's perspective and the value of patient networks, have begun to take hold, along with the emergence of more open and scalable forms of technological infrastructures to support more dispersed forms of medical assessment, treatment and service. This shift in healthcare strategy and provision is due to a number of economic, political, and socio-cultural factors, with the economic factor being predominant. The attempt to reduce the scale of healthcare expenditure has occurred through rationalizing services and shifting the burden of care from institutions back into the community. In this context, a series of new "buzzwords" have entered the healthcare discourse: patient empowerment, patient-centric perspective, self-care, mobile care, home care, patient choice, community living, ambient-assisted living, etc. Such ideas are often depicted as a panacea for many of the current problems with the inflated and over-medicalized healthcare systems in Western society.

However, along with the optimism of many about these new scenarios, including the positive contribution of technology to solving some of the problems with healthcare systems, we may also note the emergence of certain critical voices concerning this new healthcare discourse of empowerment and patient choice, and the dominant role of new technology. For instance, research on the interactions between patients and doctors in current clinical practice, consultation, and rehabilitation, has shown how the still-dominant position of the doctors and different medical experts largely limits the possibilities for patient participation and empowerment (Barry et al., 2000; Cahill, 1998; Opie, 1998), especially in chronic care (e.g. Anderson and Funnel, 2000) This paper attempts to situate the debate about new forms of augmented service delivery via technology within the larger context of the current debate about the limitations of the traditional medical model and its attendant problems in framing issues concerning self-care. We believe that discussion of new forms of augmented infrastructures does not make sense without first making explicit some of our background assumptions concerning our model of the doctor-patient relationship and the wider issues of patient self-care. At the same time, we, as researchers and designers in the area of human-machine systems, are cognizant of our limitations in the areas of medical history, political science, and economic strategy. Nevertheless, despite these shortcomings, we are of the opinion that a minimal level of under-standing of some of the issues outlined here are a prerequisite to being able to appropriately design the complex socio-technical systems that are being envisaged in the healthcare field.

INTRODUCTION

In recent years, adequate health care provision for citizens has become a major political, social, and economic concern for nation states. The increasing cost of medical infrastructures, both in administration, service delivery, and technology, is recognized as being unsustainable within the current medical model of illness prevalent in most Western countries. As a result, increasing attention has turned towards alternative, lower-cost, models of healthcare delivery. Economic arguments for healthcare reform are but one of several increasingly pressing problems with what we might term the standard healthcare model existing in Western countries. There are also major concerns among citizens with the medicalization of sickness, and with their appropriation into a logic of medicine that is often far removed from what researcher Mol has labeled the more preferable, "logic of care" (Mol, 2008).

The increasing attention to the topic of "self-care" in healthcare is brought about by the confluence of several distinct perspectives on health and illness. On the one hand, there is the clear economic motive in attempting to reduce hospital stays, and put people back into local communities and into their own homes if at all possible. There is also an empowerment motive, with the claim that self-care is required in order to ensure that people can take control of their own illness, rather than be passive consumers of a hospital-framed care model.

This issue of empowerment surfaces at many levels, from that concerned with discourse practices between doctors and patients in individual consultations, through to the feeling of helplessness induced in patents through their being shunted through a model of medical care, according to a factory-type input-output model, where patients are seen by a succession of specialists, or more usually their assistants, for very brief time periods, before being handed-off to the next "expert".

Technology also has a role to pay in this discourse, as there is an increasing interest on the part of manufacturers concerning the design and deployment of a vast array of home-health and self-care technologies into the marketplace. This upsurge is partly explained by the increasing miniaturization and decreasing cost of electronic hardware, and partly can be explained by the awareness of a huge emerging market in this sphere of home and self-care medical technologies. Coupled with an interest in the market for advanced electronic instruments, there is an increased awareness of the possibilities of networking these appliances, and thus the enrollment of these devices (& their users) into larger networked socio-technical information systems that can provide a mesh of inter-connecting services (see for instance Storni, 2010). Thus paradoxically, patients-at-home can simultaneously be seen as moving (physically) away from the geographical centre of the medical apparatus (the hospital) while, through networked home care technologies, are still actively enrolled, and in an even more comprehensive way than before, within the overall medical infrastructure.

This complex picture of healthcare trends and issues is difficult to conceptualize as a whole, but we attempt to provide some overview of the issues in Figure 1, below.

Figure 1 visually represents some of the driving entities behind the idea of self-care and the main facts, concerns, risks and opportunities that characterize their discourses (with the risk to put the patient out of focus).

In this paper, while cognizant of all of the above concerns within the current healthcare debate (Fig. 1), we focus on a subset of these myriad issues, while recognizing that it is difficult to disentangle them. The issues we discus below include: the patient-doctor relationship, the medical model of illness, patient compliance, the complex nature of infrastructures, the concept of self-care, and the role of new forms of technology within these systems, networks and infrastructure. One of the key propositions in the paper concerns the way in which, paradoxically, the call for self-care in the interests of patient empowerment can ultimately lead to new forms of enrollment of patients within a traditional medical model – this being assisted by the use of a variety of self-care medical technologies in the home. After examining and discussing this situation, we suggest a number of directions for future research and practical action that might alleviate what we believe to be a potentially troubling situation (and help to put the patient at the right focus).

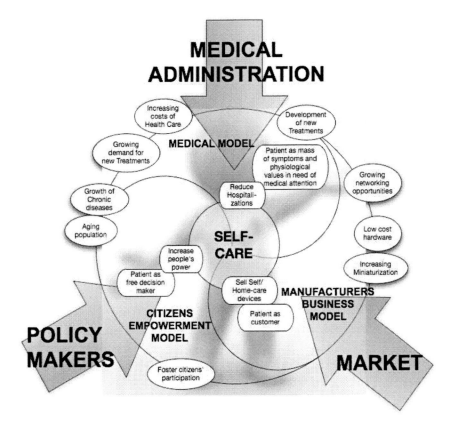

Figure 1. A representation of the complex of issues in the healthcare sector.

The paper is structured as follows: We begin with a general exploration of the standard "medical model", which deals with the evolving doctor-patent relationship over the centuries, as well as the standard medical, functional, model of illness. This raises issues such as our understanding of terms such as "being sick", and notions of (patient) compliance and empowerment. In Section 2 we provide a series of vignettes from our empirical work with doctors, pharmacists, and patients concerning self-care issues, the role of technologies, and networks of different care givers. These help to ground our discussion of issues throughout the paper. Section 3 takes up the role of technology in supporting professional practices to date, explores the issue of collaboration and the notion of infrastructure, and shows how new socio-technical infrastructuring may act as a colonizing force. Finally, in Section 4 we outline some directions for further research in both our conceptions of the healthcare system, and in the design of more open and flexible socio-technical designs.

SECTION 1 - KEY FEATURES OF THE MEDICAL MODEL

In this Section, drawing on the literature from the social study of medicine, we analyze the assumptions and connotations of the current medical model and their implications for the relationship between patients and medical experts. We first show how the "mainstream" medical model is the historical result of the consolidation and diffusion of modern medicine, producing a marked separation between the role of expert doctors and lay patients. Before describing a sampling of empirical cases, we discuss the dominant biomedical paradigm and the notion of compliance as elements that strongly characterize the current medical model.

1.1. The Role of Being a Sick Patient - In Traditional Medicine

The current separation of roles between the doctor and the sick person (patient) has become engrained in Western society with the emergence and consolidation of the medical establishment. According to Ackerknecht (1968) and Jewson (1976) (quoted in Knorr-Cetina, 1999) the early patient-doctor relationship was radically different, and was primarily based on what the authors call 'bedside science'. In the late eighteenth century and very early nineteenth century, doctors came to their patients' houses to conduct their enquiries. In this context, and with their poor equipment, the doctor's authority was extremely precarious and under scrutiny by all: family members, neighbours etc. Their weak position was due also to the way the medical examination itself was conducted. Doctors had to privilege patient's accounts and to investigate the personal and unique circumstances under which the problem occurred. This early dominance of the patient in the doctor-patient relationship changed radically with the consolidation of clinical medicine and the establishment of the biomedical paradigm in Western society.

With the birth of medical clinics (see Foucault, 1973), the relationship between the sick – now entering their modern role as 'patient' – and the expert was reversed. Patients had to leave their homes and enter a new institutionalized setting, where they would be available for observation and testing by the medical personnel. There were no family members in close proximity to sustain the patient's position, but a series of doctors collaborating to produce a diagnosis. Doctors used medical jargon, and accessed the body of the sick person through instruments that enhanced the doctors' sensory awareness over those of the patient[1]. Patients personal narratives and experiences were no longer viewed as relevant for the determination of a diagnosis. Hearing and seeing become privileged senses for the medical personnel, while medical practitioners discursive skills for interpersonal engagement with patients became devalued (Knorr-cetina, pg. 5x). In the decades after the two world wars, medicine, as Turner (1986) argues, established the social monopoly of knowledge and expertise so widely-accepted today, where patients are supposed to "fit-in" and comply with academic biomedical knowledge. Very different from the earlier 'bedside era' of medicine, the patient's knowledge and skills came to be seen as often an obstacle to the activity of doctors. Patients are expected to 'cooperate' with the doctor-prescribed therapy, in order to facilitate their reintegration into the society from which they have been temporarily excluded as a result of their medical designation of being "diseased". We will examine how more recent thinking raises some serious questions about the assumptions of this medical perspective.

1.2. Biomedical Reductionism and the Dominant Epidemiological Paradigm

Brown et al. (2006) define the normative biomedical model underpinning the dominant epidemiological paradigm. They write: *"Disease, according to this conceptual framework, is purely a biological phenomenon that can be understood through positivist, value-free research"*

This way of looking at disease – quantitative, positivistic and based on laboratory research - has important implications for the way new medical

---

[1] As Lachmund has shown (1997), the new technology of the stethoscope was tested and developed further in the new clinical setting for the exclusive use of the doctor so further privileging his position in the doctor-patient relationship.

knowledge is produced, as well as reinforcing the separation between experts (e.g. doctors) and patients. Leder (1992), who critiques biomedicine for treating the body as if it were a machine, claims:

> *"At the core of modern medical practice is the Cartesian revelation: the living body can be treated as essentially no different from a machine. [...] Insofar as the body is modeled upon a lifeless machine, the role of subjective experience in determining one's health history will tend to be overlooked".*

In this sense the patient's participation in any determination of their illness is further constrained by the doctors' belief:

> *'...that objective evidence, such as physiological indicators, or measures of functional integrity, are the only way to determine a person's health status (Molzahn, 1991) (our emphasis)*

In a scenario where self—care will become more important, Borell's concern (1993) about the role of technology in shaping the relation with the patient sounds timely:

> *"As machines provided the precision and new tests proliferated, data rather than the patient claimed the physician's attention".*

As a result,. all the practicalities, intricacies and uncertainties of dealing with a disease (especially with a chronic disease) tend to be down-played in the standard medical model. This model is also sustained by the conceptual frame that informs medical discourse. The notion of compliance in this discourse represents a paradigmatic example that deserves further attention.

1.3. Compliance in the Medical Model

Mainstream medical literature has regarded non-compliance (of patients with doctor's prescriptions) as a serious problem whose causes should be identified and remedies provided. A great deal of academic and professional effort has been devoted to developing new strategies to promote patient compliance/adherence (Anderson et al., 2000; Britten et al., 1994). This tradition reinforces the role and expertise of the professional in shaping patient behaviour. However, a small strand of sociological and anthropological studies has questioned this traditional emphasis, and instead privileges the patients' perspective (Jones, 1979; Helman, 1981; Conrad, 1985; Morgan and Watkins, 1988; Donovan, 1992; Verbeek-Heida, 1993, Robertson, 2000, Anderson et al. 2000, Osterberg and Blaschke, 2005). According to this alternative view, autonomous patients will develop their own medication practice (especially in the context of chronic disease), even though this may not coincide with the institutionalized health professionals' recommendations. Much of this behavior could be seen as non-compliance, but, from the patient's perspective, it is not[2]. Pioneering this perspective, Conrad (1985) articulates:

> 'the whole notion of compliance suggests a medically-centered orientation; how and why people follow or deviate from doctor's orders. It is a concept developed from the doctor's perspective and conceived to solve the provider-defined problem of 'noncompliance'. The assumption is the doctor gives the orders; patients are expected to comply. It is based on a consensual model of doctor-patient relations, aligning with Parsons' perspective, where noncompliance is deemed a form of deviance in need of explanation.

Conrad studied people with epilepsy. Using a commonly accepted criterion for measuring compliance, he found that 42 percent of respondents could be seen as non-compliant. Yet from a patient's perspective the issues are not about complying or not complying. For instance, most of the people with chronic disease spend only a tiny fraction of their lives in the traditional 'patient role'.

> 'Embedded in the context of their own experience, their use of medications can better be seen as a form of "self-regulation." [...] Compliance assumes that the doctor-patient relationship is pivotal for subsequent action, which may not be the case[3]. (Ibid)

---

[2] Similarly, Robertson (1992) shows how the doctor and the patient display a different understanding of compliance. What the doctor sees as non-compliant behavior is often understood as 'doing a pretty good job' by patients.

[3] Also focusing on diabetes, general practitioners Anderson and Funnell (2000) argue that the problem arises due to the inappropriate use of a traditional acute care model for the case of chronic diseases: 'The resolution lies in the recognition that as healthcare professionals we have been socialized to a set of needs, beliefs, and methods that may work reasonably well in the treatment of acute illness but are fundamentally unworkable in diabetes care.' [...] 'what we are suggesting is that we need a new conceptual framework for self-management behaviour of the patient and our role and relationship with patients'

In this sense, the notion of compliance acts as another strategy of exclusion of the experience of the patient through its often paternalistic and coercive assumptions. According to Osterberg and Blaschke (2005), both of the terms, compliance and adherence, are imperfect and uninformative descriptions of medication-taking behaviour in self-care. They argue for the need to reassess these terms as they are still dominant in medical practice and result in patients being blamed, (for not being compliant) or even, on occasion, doctors themselves! (for being insensitive to personal issues that prevent compliance).

Summary

This brief and partial outline of the literature on the evolution of what is now termed the standard medical model, and the diminution of the patient's voice, is noted here due to its importance in understanding the current situation in which we find ourselves. The ideal of the patient as a more active partner in their interaction with the doctor is more difficult to achieve than it might at first seem. We also wish to show how the underlying medical model has enrolled new technologies into its ambit, even in the context of the supposedly changed discourse around healthcare delivery, self-care and patient empowerment. In the next section we provide evidence from our initial empirical investigations of what are termed "self-care" practices and technology. Despite the language of patient empowerment often associated with self-care initiatives, and the supportive role of new technologies in this changed set of practices, we show that the same difficulties mentioned above are also found in these self-care practices.

Our focus here is on two particular kinds of self-care technology and practices: blood pressure monitors (BPM) and glucose meters (GM), that support self-monitoring in two of the most widespread and worrying chronic diseases: cardiovascular diseases such as *hypertension,* and *diabetes.* We show how complex the issue of self-care is and how the traditional characteristics of the medical model might become problematic when uncritically extended, from traditional institutionalized settings and expert users, to new emerging settings and lay users.

SECTION 2 - SELF-CARE PRACTICES AND TECHNOLOGY: CASES FROM SELF-MONITORING

Our focus on self-monitoring devices is motivated by the fact that these devices are being manufactured and "consumed" at an exponential rate[4]. It is also the case that these devices, while often currently of a "stand-alone" type, will soon become networked into larger healthcare technical infrastructures. Thus the reach of the technical medical infrastructure can be extended into the home and the body of the patient, even while the patient is no longer under the direct institutional surveillance of the medical system (e.g. in a hospital setting). This scenario, of the extension of the medical infrastructure into the personal living space of the patient via the utilization of new self-care technologies, raises a number of troubling questions for us – in the context of improving the doctor-patient relation and producing more favorable health outcomes for the patient in these "augmented" care settings. Let us examine some of these situations as we have encountered them in our field studies.

2.1. Vignette 1: An Elderly Woman Has Problems with a Blood Pressure Monitor

This first vignette is extracted from an interview with a general practitioner. The interview investigated the GP's interaction with patients and, more specifically, the problems the GP has experienced with patients

---

[4] Recent research from MINTEL show that sales of self-diagnostics in UK has grown by 40% since 2000 and will rise by a further 38% by 2010. Sales of Blood pressure monitors have almost doubled in value from 2002 to 2004. The number of adults monitoring their blood pressure has increased by 250% from 1999 to 2008. A companion report - "The Consumer Medical Production Yearbook", from InMedica (IMS' medical electronics division) - forecasts exceptional growth in consumer medical devices with manufacturer revenues reaching over $5 billion by 2011. Looking to the future, MINTEL predicts a staggering 60% increase in the market of blood pressure, blood glucose and body fat measuring kits to 2012, with sales expected to reach £158 million, as growing awareness of health issues fuel sales of self diagnostics. For more detailed information visit:
http://www.marketresearchworld.net/index.php?option=com_content&task=view&id=400&Itemid=77;
http://www.marketresearchworld.net/index.php?option=com_content&task=view&id=1912&Itemid=77;
http://www.marketresearchworld.net/index.php?option=com_content&task=view&id=1668&Itemid=77.

difficulties with self-monitoring activities and technology in their own home spaces.

> *Brian, general practitioner: With one particular lady, we were having difficulties controlling her blood pressure. ... Her blood pressure was not controlled anyway, but we were compromising because we were controlling her blood pressure when she started having episodes of postural blood pressure drop ... when she was going from sitting to standing she got dizzy and so she was in danger and at risk of falling..... . This lady is 80 years of age ... so we decided to have her blood pressure run a little bit higher. So instead of running at 148 ... we tried to set it at 155 - 160 by giving her fewer pills so that her blood pressure would be a little bit higher ... and she was feeling better and we were adjusting other factors as she was on aspirin to minimize her risk of stroke ... but then she started getting some really high readings on her own device; she was measuring her blood pressure six, seven times a day ... completely over the top and sometimes she was getting a reading of 240 and 120 ... even though most of her readings were about 150 to 170 or maybe 90 to 95 ... She was also getting these particular readings really high ... so she started to measure her blood pressure even more often, 10, 12 times a day ... and she was not sleeping at night and she was convinced that she was going to have a stroke any minute ... and she got so bad that we eventually had to admit her to the hospital because she was so absolutely out ... and when she came home from the hospital she was a lot better.... She was happy that she had not had any heart attacks; she was happy that she had not had a stroke but she was still afraid she was going to get one ... so I had to tranquillize her, give her enough tranquilizers so that she was sleeping at night ... and I had to keep her that way for two weeks and I had to keep her blood pressure monitor away from her.... It took about a month to get back to a state when she could live by herself,... She went totally nuts ...*
> *ME: Is she living alone?*
> *GP: No, she is living with her blind husband ...*

Although this vignette might appear quite extreme, based on our investigations, we believe it is not that unusual. Almost all the health care professionals we interviewed[5] seemed familiar with this kind of problem and

---

[5] The data set is based on a series of in-depth interviews with Italian and Irish Health Care professionals (such as General practitioners and community pharmacists) and chronic disease patient (such as Diabetes type 1 and hypertension patients), and session of ethnographic observations (in community pharmacies) and a self-support group for individuals with diabetes type 1. Three Italian pharmacists were interviewed for 40, 45 and 100 minutes respectively. Three Irish pharmacists were interviewed for 80, 90 and 75

mentioned many similar instances, as the next series of extracts from interviews with three Italian community pharmacists reaffirms:

Giulia, Pharmacist: People come in twice and more ... they are afraid to make mistakes. When test results vary a lot, they come back here and ask if they perform the test correctly, if the device works properly; they ask if they can double check with my machine here in the shop...

Lorenzo, Pharmacist: Elderly people in particular have problems. They buy these machines and then they come back because they start to test themselves continuously.... So while you have some patients that start using them correctly, some elderly people just go mad with these things ...

Guido, Pharmacist: One day, an old woman did many tests and she brought the device back to the shop because she got too many different results. This has also to do with their expectations. People say: It is morning, I have not done anything particular, I am home and I feel fine. Why should I have changes in my blood pressure?

This series of extracts illustrate quite clearly that in their use of blood-pressure monitors, patients (especially, but not only, elderly people) develop a series of *problematic testing practices* that complicate rather than ease their relationship with the doctors, and the management of their therapy. Whether it is uncertainty about the proper use of the device or anxiety about high readings, the core of these practices relies on the interaction between patients and biomedical test results (numbers), and on the patients' ability to make sense of them. When this interaction becomes problematic, the appropriation of self-monitoring devices does not lead to purported patient empowerment, but rather results in blind dependencies on readings whose meaning might be difficult to grasp and whose validity is doubtful.

Take the above initial example by the general practitioner Brian. Here we have a patient who has been equipped with a self-monitoring device because

minutes respectively. One Irish pharmacist preferred not to be recorded. Two general practitioners and one specialist (one Italian and two Irish) were interviewed for 90 and 100 minutes. Diabetes patients (9 Irish and 3 Italian) were interviewed averagely for 90 minutes. Reported names are purely fictional. Interviews were informal, open and unstructured although a series of general topics were repeatedly discussed. Interviews with professionals were open and with a particular emphasis on their problematic relations with patients or on aspects concerning the use of medical technology, the management of emergencies, self-care and self-medication practices. Chronic disease patients were interviewed extensively regarding their daily dealing with the disease, their relationships with medical personnel and the pro and contras of using self care technology. Interviewees were constantly invited to provide practical examples and stories instead of talking in general terms.

the GP needs to monitor certain parameters in order to adjust the woman's therapy (something quite common in our aging society). However, once left alone in the context of her domestic environment, this attempt to provide the patient with a limited autonomy generated the following litany of additional problems: an extra hospitalization, the need to use tranquilizers, and the fact that the originally intended cure had to be postponed by one month (not to mention that the patient had to take care of her blind husband)! What results from this episode is an increase in healthcare costs, and an obstruction of the potential to learn about the disease – on the part of both the doctor (who has to deal with unreliable data) and the patient (who has to deal with her own inability to use the device and make sense of the results).

2.2. Vignette 2: Marc, the Autonomous Diabetic Patient

Marc was diagnosed with diabetes type 1 when he was 15 years old. He is 34 now. He recalls his experience as almost traumatic because he suddenly found himself

> *Marc: ...catapulted into a strict regime of diet – which is not just eating with moderation, but more specifically not eating specific things - and injections ... I recall at the beginning, it was all about making holes and injections. Nobody really explained to me what was going on if not just the very basics, such as, 'You should not eat this and that; you should do these injections.' That is it. Nobody talked about glucose, how insulin is supposed to interact and stuff like that ... .I only got a leaflet for the diet showing the amount of carbs in common food.... At the time, we did not have the Internet; there was no Wikipedia or users' online forums.*

After almost 20 years of dealing with diabetes type 1, Marc had slowly gained control of the disease by a series of what he called 'trials and corrections', through which he also learned to better make sense of his bodily sensations. More specifically, Marc had come to distinguish two different aspects of measuring glucose levels at home, which represent two different forms of self-empowerment with the glucose meter.

> *Marc: I think I see two aspects of self-measurement. The first is to check your level with respect to a value that you know you should try to keep stable: this is a sort of fetish, is what your doctor asks you to do.... The second is a sort of verification when you do not feel well and you want to see if that depends on your level of glucose, in case you can*

intervene by eating something or by getting some extra insulin units.... So, home measurements have also this kind of emergency and self-understanding function, that is, to see if your feeling dizzy depends on your blood level or on something else.... This is very useful ...

When asked about the role of the doctor in this self-management practice, Marc reaffirmed that he has now achieved total autonomy in his self-care.

Marc: I completely manage my therapy myself.... I do not have any interaction with the GP on this aspect.... I do it myself also because you come to realize that the GP cannot follow all your specific problems, moreover they do not know much about living with diabetes... so what happens is that you make some sort of mental plans by yourself... something like: I read 200 with the meter, if I do 2 units of insulin I will go to 120, with 3 units I will be around 80 and so on ... [Interviewer: Well, yes, I see, but then you start to include elements of your life in these mental plans ... right?] Certainly! Every time, I make a plan depending on where I am, what I am supposed to do, and it changes according to the fact that I am at home, in the office or not, whether I can prepare my food or just get something from a menu.... For instance, when I know we are going to be walking for a long time because we are sightseeing somewhere or we are in the countryside, I tend to keep my level of glucose a little higher, so instead of 10 units of insulin before lunch, I take only 9 or 8.... If I know I will have a football match to play I will do even fewer units... Of course, at the beginning, you give it a try and you see what happens, but without self-measurement and the meter you cannot even think of doing these things ... and, more importantly, nobody teaches you this ...

When Marc was first diagnosed, he was concerned with understanding how to behave properly, to use the equipment the way it is supposed to be used and, basically, to survive. Self-care for him was trying to behave in accordance with what the GP and the specialist prescribed. Through the accumulation of experiences in the form of personal trials, errors and corrections, which lasted for years, *his relationship with the disease and with the equipment changed.* Initially, the glucose meter was used to comply with the doctor's advice and to try to keep the glucose level stable at a certain level, which Marc defined as a *fetish.* With time, the meter became entangled with the intricacies of Marc's life and its use became progressively intertwined within an entire series of everyday practices, such as doing physical exercise, eating out and so on. The use of the glucose meter moved from a situation where it reinforced the ideal nature of the biomedical optimal level of sugar in the blood to a situation within which the optimal level of glucose was not an *absolute academic value* (e.g., 100 mg/dl), but rather a *practical value* related to Marc's self-management (e.g., 120/140 if he wants to run a bit after lunch). Now, its use goes beyond the simple measurement activity or compliance, but is a form of autonomous self-regulation to adjust the intake to unique, personal and often unplanned activities; and more interestingly, the doctor is no longer in the picture.

The next series of extracts show some similarities with the case of Marc but further illustrate how the separation between the "patient" and the doctor can exacerbate into an open conflict.

> **Paula**: *'it is hard to find a specialist who acknowledges that the patient knows just as much, here it is always the opinion: "ok I am the doctor you are the stupid patient, you do what I tell you..." but that's not right! A diabetic needs to be an endocrinologist, a sports adviser, a nutritionist. You need to be all that in one person in order to deal with your diabetes but doctors don't understand [...] They think you are stupid, they don't realize that you think about what you are doing because they don't live with it, they don't see the numbers they just read it on paper, they go home at night and eat their dinner and don't think about carbohydrates and the whole lot'.*

In talking about her attempt to build a constructive relationship with her endocrinologist, especially concerning her will to self-adjust the regime of insulin, Paula underlined:

> **Paula:** *'She didn't really see it as a problem as such, but on the other side how could she? She's not living with it, she only sees it on paper! she doesn't live with diabetes! It's completely different...so sometimes doctors can't relate to your concern in a certain problem because they just don't have it'.*

As clearly explained by another patient:

> **Gabriela:** *In order to get proper care you have to start test or training the doctors.*

In particular Gabriela discussed how the metric of compliance and the intrinsic biomedical reductionism of the medical understanding of the disease affect the interaction with the medical expert. Indeed, this conflict can grow, to a point when the patient might even start to hide things to better comply with the doctor's expectations. In talking about the need to keep track of different 'lay' aspects of their life she said:

> **Gabriela**: *I type those [extra information] out for my doctor because if I handed that to her she would be like, what is this?? So she has a format where I just put in the numbers, I just put in the readings and the units. That's all! she doesn't want to know anything else. [...] she's not really doing her job properly she doesn't look at what I eat. [...] Some doctors would make judgements on one reading.*

As tests proliferate, these additional "objective" measures will further drawn the attention of the expert away from the needed further dialogue with the patient who – especially now with the availability of support through the Internet, health social networks and support groups – will be likely to supplement, or even replace, the medical advice with other community advice. This is clearly shown in the extract below:

> **Geraldine**: *You don't want to seem stupid for suggesting something that the doctor is going to turn around and say: 'no, that's not relevant'. You might think you are learning all these new things and you think they're relevant but if she's not open to it then your not going to be forthcoming...that's what's missing from that side...well, we make up for it!*

The problem here is not making up for the lack of dialogue, but the fact that doctors may not be aware of the source and variety of advice that an individual with a chronic disease may receive, assuming that they are the only advice givers of relevance to the patient.

As mentioned, compliance is often not the main problem for the patient. Patients may need to solve a problem that a particular drug or procedure creates in their life by developing their own network of care givers, even if this might not coincide with the institutionalized one. In the most disturbing cases we have witnessed, patients find themselves viewing the doctor as an adversary: someone either to ignore or to blame.

On examining the current trend to send patients back to their homes, where they are supported by the increasing diffusion of a variety of self-care and home-care technology (monitoring devices that constantly produce a stream of numerical data, implants, therapeutic and self-medication devices, technical aids, public information repositories, etc.), we find that the idea of an emancipated patient, empowered by this self-care technology enveloping them, is often a myth.

Think of the use of the glucose meter in Marc's case. What if the glucose meter was part of a larger infrastructure allowing the doctors to monitor Marc's activities? In a world with an increasing number of individuals with chronic disease and the mass diffusion of self-monitoring devices, there is a danger that there will be a further increase in the doctor-patient divide. As self-care increases, the current medical model and its logics are likely to afford either worrying interactions - because patients are not able to self-regulate safely (as in the case of the elderly lady) -, or conflicts - because they feel the system fails to address the unique and holistic circumstances of a particular individual (as in the case of Marc, but alo Paula and Gabriela). The former interactions generate a set of concerns for those patients who have difficulties in relating to the biomedical domain and for whom self-care and empowerment often means "getting lost" or confused. The latter interactions tend to develop antagonistic perspectives that constrain the dialogue between patients and doctors (either because the patient stops going to the doctor, or because the patient gives up arguing with the doctors). In both cases, what is really compromised is any chance for *mutual learning* and the possibility of creating room for further dialogue - to explore viable solutions together. By fostering antagonistic and asymmetrical dialogues that are often afforded and re-produced by the way we conceive self-care technology, these worrying interactions and conflicts threaten the very idea of addressing current healthcare issues with self-care.

We believe that a central issue here is the separation between the idea of educating the patient and that of disciplining the patient. This confusion surfaces at many levels in the discussed vignettes. We, as designers and developers of solutions for the patient, cannot expect them to be necessarily literate and unproblematically relate with the biomedical perspective and the idea of compliance (as in the case of the elderly lady). At the same time we cannot expect biomedical knowledge to be the only one available to influence the patient's behaviour (as in the case of Marc whose lay expertise goes beyond a literal application of a biomedical prescription) as well as to improve health outcomes. The risk is in fact to create worries in those who do not understand enough, and *wars* with those who develop their own autonomy to better deal with the unique aspect of their disease in everyday life. In both cases disciplining and colonizing the patient view with a top-down infrastructure does not seem to be the answer we need. We believe that a possible answer should be found in the way we think of collaboration between patient and their care-givers, and what sort of health infrastructure can support this. For this purpose we now pass to those studies that have put the role of technology in supporting collaboration at the centre, as well as studies that have addressed the role of infrastructure in shaping our socio-technical systems.

SECTION 3 - HEALTH AND ICT, ON COLLABORATION AND E-HEALTH INFRASTRUCTURES

In this Section we provide a number of arguments as to how our current perspective on healthcare delivery, supported with technology, is limiting, and needs to be re-considered in the light of some of the issues we have described. We organize our arguments around a set of topics - the role of technology in professional practice, the discussion on infrastructures and their intrinsic need to "freeze" emerging practices.

3.1. CSCW – Traditional Support for Expert Socio-Technical Practices

The empirical investigation of complex professional settings such as hospitals, with a view to understanding how the activities of the professionals may be supported via various technological infrastructures, has grown rapidly in recent years. Much, though not all, of this work has been conducted through various forms of ethnographic investigations. Such workplace studies have often been presented at Computer Supported Cooperative Work conferences, where there is a strong interest in the coordination and collaboration mechanisms uncovered, and how they might be supported with technologies. Thanks to the work of a number of scholars we have come to understand some of the subtleties of communication, coordination and collaboration practices of medical experts in their specialized workplaces (Berg, 1999; Wintbereik and Vikkelso, 2005; Schmidt and Simone, 1996). We have developed an understanding of the role of material settings, artifacts, and inscriptions (Suchman, 1994; Ellingsen et al., 2006); standards and classifications (Bowker and Star, 2000; Hanseth at al. 1993); and the distribution of activities in hospital wards (Berg, 1999; Berg and Timmermans, 2000), clinics, and laboratories (Jirotka et al. 2005). We have discovered how the circulation of information in work settings can be problematic, as meaning is situated, and a deep understanding of specific contexts is vital (Winthereik and Vikkelso, 2005; Ure et al. 2009). The focus of all of these studies is on the circulation of expert knowledge (as in Jirotka et al. 2005; Martin et al. 2006; Procter et al. 2006) and in the understanding of expert practices in professional environments (as in Berg, 1999; Fitzpatrick, 2004; Reddy et al. 2006; Schneider and Wagner, 1993 and many others). All of these detailed and insightful studies explore the perspectives of various professional groups and discuss how these expert practices might be augmented through technologies. Concepts such as shared-care, integrated care, and continuity of care, have become cornerstones in the drive to develop and implement coherent, dependable, seamless, integrated and effective healthcare systems and services (Procter et al. 2006; Elligsen and Monteiro, 2006). Another of the key orienting concepts for researchers in healthcare technology and collaborative professional practice (as well as this special issue) is that of "infrastructure" – at both a technical and organizational level (see Edwards et al. 2009).

3.2. Infrastructures and Infrastructuring

The aim of studies on infrastructure varies – from a focus on defining what infrastructures are (Star and Ruhleder, 1996), to how they can be studied (Star, 1999), to how they can be better designed and implemented (e.g. Turner et al. 2006, Star and Bowker, 2002; and Hanset et Braa, 2001). Many of these studies also address issues of maintenance and the need for continuous adjustment and improvement in the infrastructuring process (e.g. Hanset and Lundberg, 2001).

We have learned that infrastructures are embedded and transparent; that they go beyond a single event and become visible upon breakdown (Star and Ruhleder, 1996). We also have learned that they link with pre-existing conventions, that they build on an installed base, and that they embed standards. This latter aspect is often seen as an essential feature of an infrastructure. Star and Bowker (2002) write:

> "...both standardization and classification are essential to the development of working infrastructure...[...] people's discursive and work practices get hustled into standard form as well. Working infrastructures standardize both people and machines..."

Now, given that infrastructure is built upon existing practices, it is clear that the establishment of a standard will unavoidably change some of these practices and privilege certain aspects to the detriment of others. The authors mention the '*relative usefulness of infrastructures for different populations of users*' showing that the notion of infrastructure is not absolute but relative to working conditions (Start and Bowker, 2002). Again, Ribes and Finhalt (2009) warn against marginalizing participants in what they call *the long now* of an infrastructure, a notion that challenges the short orientation of early infrastructure studies. Their concern is that - once the infrastructure has been settled - future uses might be severely constrained by embedded decisions that indeed take the form of standards, classifications and formalized procedures.

This problem is so common in the emerging field of infrastructure studies that authors deal with it in different ways. Talking of design of infrastructure, Star and Bowker (2002), for instance, conclude that: *the work of design is in many ways secondary to the work of modification...* and that *...Infrastructure subtends complex ecologies: their design process should always be tentative, flexible and open'*. Other authors reaffirm this. Focusing on the implementation phases, Hanseth and Braa, for instance, showed how a *Universal* (e.g. a standard) never gets implemented as such: "*its universal character disappears during implementation*" (2001) because it adapts to local circumstances. Pipek and Wulf (2009), show that users will inevitably re-shape a new infrastructure during use and should always be considered "designers". To reinforce this position and escape the standardizing nature of infrastructure they use Star's notion of *infrastructur-ing* that underlines the need to keep the infrastructure open to user appropriation. Earlier, Hanseth et al. (1993) discussed a series of strategies for dealing with issues of centralization, standardization and formalization intrinsic to the design and implementation of infrastructures by concluding that the design and implementation should be always *participatory and evolutionary*.

However, although Star & Bowker (2002) have suggested a distinction between a colonial model and a democratic model of infrastructure, the notion of infrastructure with its standardizing logic can be viewed as intrinsically colonial for many of its users. This is because the infrastructure will eventually be "frozen" in a certain fashion, at a specific time, thus unavoidably privileging some actors and their practices and perspectives over the others. The ideal of a centralizing control model, as outlined in Ciborra and Hanseth

(1998), proliferates, and infrastructures tend to become dominating super-structures, with a unified language and a form of centralized control[6].

It follows from this discussion that the notion of infrastructure displays two essential and at the same time highly problematic characteristics, from our point of view: its non-neutrality toward different populations of users, and the consequent and unavoidable problematic nature of its implementation, where different actors struggle against the totalizing infrastructural frame of the privileged discourse. In the healthcare sector, these are two core problems, especially in the context of the current debates about home care and self-care technologies. We have seen how the biomedical standard operate a form of epistemological reductionism that often marginalizes the participation of patients if not even generate conflicts and barriers to much-needed colla-borations. We can see this also operating in our vignettes. Our concern here is that discussion about healthcare infrastructure might simply end up privileging the dominant paradigm by magnifying and not reducing the conflictual nature of the relationship between patients (who know their disease *in-the-wild* through their subjective experience) and experts (who know the disease *in-vitro* in theoretical biomedical terms). The risk is to assume that infrastructures should support those who should know what is best for the patient (the doctor's perspective) and provide support for their work so that the benefits will (it is assumed) accrue to the patient. What is worrying is that often in discussions of improving healthcare support systems, there is little mention of any role for the patient. For example, Pinelle et al. state:

> *"One of the main promises of CSCW technologies in healthcare is to improve the dependability of the care delivery process – by improving patient safety, by improving the overall responsiveness of the healthcare organization, or by improving the overall effectiveness of care delivery. By improving the flow of information within the organization, and by improving overall information access by practitioners and key decision makers, these technologies have the potential to improve the overall level of care that is provided to patients"*

We think that this might be a rather limited idea especially if confronted with new domestic environments where people ("patients") are themselves using self-care technology. Indeed, what is striking here (and in the literature we have reviewed at the beginning of this section) is that despite the large

---

[6] Brown and Duguid (2000) and Bowker and Star (2000) have underlined the social and often political nature of the collection, classification, and representation of information.

number of thoughtful research projects carried out in healthcare settings mentioned at the beginning of this section, the focus on the patient as one of the key decision-makers involved and their perspective is rarely mentioned! The problem is therefore that the emergence of pervasive computerized and networked environments supporting self-care may end up facilitating the implementation of the privileged set of medical cultural values and perspectives rather than opening up new spaces to take into account the heterogeneity of the patient population. Thus the notion of infrastructure in a deep sense presupposes some form of homogeneity. More than something "below" (its etymological sense) it suggests something on "top" – a superstructure: on top of everybody, the same for everybody.

In sum, in our view, the language of infrastructures is too deterministic – it suggests a model where different populations of users get irreversibly enrolled, (railroaded, framed) into the same program, within the same perspective, and under the same dominant language and the same set of pre-figured concerns. It supports the notion that those who are attached to the infrastructure (e.g. their blood pressure monitor has been networked, and their data is uploaded automatically and continuously to the clinic) become part of a system where the power, the procedures and the language have already been irreversibly fixed. It suggests a framing process where patients are somehow co-opted into a pre-defined solution[7]. The idea of e-health infrastructure is not adequate to acknowledge the variety of user populations in health care. We have talked about the patient, but who is the patient? We have young and old people, we have acute and chronic diseases, some of them are severely symptomatic and impairing, some others not, thus making the experience of living with the disease rather different. We have enormous geographical differences, socio-economical conditions and cultural milieus. A patient-centric perspective should be based on appreciating this variety while the notion of infrastructure and the traditional focus on the collaboration between 'experts' do not seem to help. As Goguen claims (2005), we need to support diversity and not suppress it. And this is especially true when it comes to uncertainties, and medicine – despite the impressive achievements of the past century - is still an uncertain domain[8].

---

[7] Hence users may become producers, but they do not own the language or the means of communication or dissemination of their "labour", but rather have their output inscribed in the corpus of the patient record system, which is not even always directly available to the client/patient!

[8] Turner et al. (2006) have argued that pre-formatting an environment only works in situations where the environment is stable. In health care this logic cannot work simply because the

In short, we believe that the notion of infrastructure obfuscates rather than clarifies the idea of empowering patients and self-care. We need instead to rethink the relationship between patients and experts across all our complex socio-technical healthcare systems. We rather think that the field of infrastructure studies in the medical domain needs to extend its reach to settings that involve more heterogeneity (or hybridity) both in terms of the actors and the languages that are crucially involved, and the settings where the action takes place.

3.3. Re-Thinking Empowerment: A Critical Look at the Notion of Self in Self-Care

The idea of patients that are empowered because doctors and developers provide them with some limited agency contradicts the basic principle of empowerment, which is that it is something that one takes on oneself, not something that is given to one. This false notion of empowerment disguises the fact that underneath the rhetoric, the dominant model of power relations and privileged discourse remains unchallenged, especially with the consolidating role of e-health infrastructure that reproduce the traditional assumptions. The question thus becomes: who is allowed to define what empowerment means? – Experts trapped in a biomedical understanding of the disease or patients themselves, first-in-line in dealing with the disease itself? Or why not both of them, as cooperating parties engaged in an open-ended negotiation?

One of the things that we believe should be addressed - before we start to enroll a huge variety of patients into health care infrastructures (through silent *wi-fi tentacles* reaching into domestic environments) is the complexity of the notion of "patient" and its implications for what we mean by "self" in self-care. Self-care should not be understood as an individual activity, despite the language of the Self that is used as a banner[9]. There is always a collective or a coalition of assemblies behind what looks like an individual or an individual

---

Health environment is anything but stable, especially when patients are enrolled in self-care technologies: diseases in-the-wild are entangled with social elements in the domestic environment, they are multi-facetted, and complex, and there is no fixed classification, or formalization that can easily cope with such heterogeneity.

[9] Of course, there are a few unfortunate people who live totally alone, but even in these cases self-care is not just about isolated, individual, activities. Patients belong to families and extended relation networks, they have workmates, friends, people they know, in the places they visit.

action; and this principle does not change for self-care. Patients are what they are and do what they do *in relation to* and *within,* a series of collectives. In this sense, the patient's good health and well-being cannot be understood as attributes of a more or less "bio-medically" empowered individual but rather as what is produced and reproduced within a series of overlapping collectives. These collectives are heterogeneous in nature (because they are both social and technical) and hybrid (because lay perspectives co-exists with expert ones). Here different networks of entities are mobilized through a series of practices that encounter, get along, struggle, and influence one another.

This position is articulated most clearly in the careful elaboration by Mol (2008), who has critiqued the dominant rational model underlying the notion of patient choice (a notion which again aligns with the traditional medical model and implies a self-bounded and self-responsible individual). Mol presents her argument in the context of 2 distinct logics – a logic of Choice, and a logic of Care. The Logic of Choice assumes that we are separate individuals who form a collective when we are added together. In the logic of care by contrast,

> *"we do not start out as individual, but always belong to a collective already - and not just a single one, but a lot of them..."(Mol, 2008)*

This perspective enriches our view of the vignettes we presented earlier. In our second vignette, Marc's experiment to gain autonomy in managing his disease comes from encounters with those who have already been there. The same can be said for the other diabetics, who meet once a week with a group of patients with the same disease to exchange tips and comfort one another. The same thing can be also said for the woman in Vignette 1 whose preoccupations were probably amplified by the need to be present and active enough for her blind and older husband.

But recently the collective that makes up the identity and agency of the patient are also changing. For instance, patients today start to look for those who share the same conditions and form support groups. With the advent of the Internet, email, interest groups, and social software, the possibilities for engaging with like-minded others, people who share illnesses, concerns, worries etc., have enlarged considerably. The growth of such self-care communities has been phenomenal (Preece, 1998; Kamel Boulos et al. 2007; Nettleton and Burrows, 2003; Hardey, 2001). Some join patient online communities such as www.patientslikeme.com or patients' blogs such as www.diabetesmine.com. Some of them look for information or confirmation while some others lead discussions and produce information and narratives[10]. New forms of collaborations are already there too. Think of the role that certain patient associations are playing in the shaping of the identity of patients and in the production of medical knowledge and clinical trials. A corpus of recent literature on patient associations explores patient participation at a more collective level and shows how alternative languages, ways of looking at the disease, and relating with the traditional medical *status quo* are possible (Barbot, 2006; Brown et al., 2006; Callon et al. 2009, Rabeharisoa and Callon, 1998, 2004). For instance, Barbot (2006) studied the history of a series of AIDS patient associations. She distinguished a series of ways in which these associations redefine patient participation: *patients as managers of their disease* with emphasis on the problem of patient marginalization; patients as *empowered sufferer* with a critique of the medical model that disregards patient experience; *science-wise patients* who wish to take part in cutting edge research; and *patients as experimenters* who create their own research agenda and conduct their own experiments. These models are also discussed, in similar terms, by Brown et al. (2006) who distinguish three different levels of patient participation: doing scientific research, interpreting science and acting on science. In their interesting analysis of controversies on breast cancers they show how laypeople and activists have generated new medical knowledge[11] while erasing lay-expert boundaries and transporting science into public spheres for public use[12]. The recent emergence of Bio-hacker spaces further extends the range of new ways in which medical expert knowledge and different perspectives can enrich one another and not necessarily clash.

In sum, we believe that the language of "self-care" needs to be treated with caution as it tends to overemphasize the notion of the responsible individual and downplays other perspectives viz., on the one hand, the very conception of an autonomous individual entity, a conception that is open to

---

[10] see Hardey (2001) who addresses the role of the Internet in the birth of what he calls the Informed patient - who not only consumes but also produces health information. This is seen as threatening the traditional medical status quo.

[11] An example of this kind of lay produced science is the Cape Cod Breast Cancer and Environment study Atlas which contains Cape-specific information on breast cancer incidence, historical pesticide use, drinking-water quality, census data, and land use such as the location of waste-disposal sites and the dramatic transition from forested land to residential housing.

[12] The role of lay people in the production and dissemination of scientific knowledge has been previously addressed by Callon and his associates (Callon, 1999, Rabeharisoa and Callon, 1998, 2004). Their research shows that laypeople can contribute to the existing body of medical knowledge, complementing and integrating it, but also bitterly contesting it, as in the case presented by Arksay and Sloper (1999).

serious critique, and on the other, the realization that in our society few people really function as completely autonomous individuals; rather they are multiply enrolled in a variety of larger groupings of couples, partners, families, relations, clubs, groups, etc...which all can have a significant bearing on conceptualizing "self-care" practices and "self-care" technologies.

3.4. Summary

The extension of self-care technology into domestic environments has been heralded as opening up new vistas, not only in affording more effective healthcare management, but also in patient/customer empowerment and convenience. However, we have argued that the more likely scenario of such a deployment – in the current climate – is an extension of the dominant medical model of illness further into the everyday lives of the patient, resulting in further strengthening the passive role of the patient, who is now increasingly having their behaviour and vital signs monitored and recorded through the use of pervasive personal and domestic technologies. Our concern here is not simply to replace one dominant model with another, but rather to attempt to ensure that alternative models, especially those that provide a voice for the patient/user/consumer, are not eliminated from consideration from the outset.

There is a danger of these new systems marginalizing, not so much patients *per se,* but more specifically the possibility of alternative ways of knowing and dealing with disease to the detriment of collective learning. Nowadays patients rarely feel in control of what is going on with their health and too often experience extremely problematic and painful treatment trajectories. Our case regarding Marc – the experienced diabetic patient – shows that as people gain sufficient knowledge to self-manage, they may just unplug from the enframing systems and disappear from medical attention. From their perspective, such behaviour shows a real sense of empowerment, and allows them to confront a system where their doctors '*cannot understand*', and who '*only looks at numbers*' as also shown.

The encounter of Health Care infrastructure with that of patient empowerment and self-care thus might end up creating a paradox: patients supposedly empowered and enabled to take care of themselves through a form of delegation ultimately find themselves, at another level, enrolled into the larger, and more traditional, health care infrastructures. This inclusion might then operate a silent exclusion of their perspective through the imposition of a biomedical language and specific way of looking at things. The result would be that of giving the patient a voice in order to better (and remotely) silence and discipline them. As we noted in the discussion of the infrastructure literature, a form of colonialism is almost inevitable, so is it any wonder if we are confronted with research studies that show local struggles over ownership of information, representational formats, and their meanings, and the need for expensive continuous adjustments and modifications to these monochrome infrastructures. Our research shows that if we move too quickly and too directly toward infrastructur-ing self care with the idea of empowering patients, some of them will simply rebel by disappearing from the system, some will develop frantic practices and much frustration, while many others will continue to struggle with their chronic disease because empowerment for them means being left alone, or blamed, if something goes wrong.

SECTION 4 - IMPLICATIONS FOR PATIENT-CENTRIC DESIGN

We believe that the series of arguments we have collected have important design implications for health care in general, and self-care in particular. They allow us to explore alternatives and to start asking questions regarding the role of the patient, their ways of experiencing and knowing their disease, their interaction with medical technology and professionals and, consequently, the role of design and technology in patient health. In this concluding section we briefly introduce a general design principle and outline certain themes that may support the creation of spaces for dialogue between different perspectives on disease, and support the collective experimentation and tuning of care. These spaces and socio-technical support platforms may remove the strong asymmetry that currently exists between the patient and medical experts that hinder mutual collaboration.

4.1. The Problem of "Fixing Things" - The Need for On-Going Openness and Flexibility in the Act of Categorization

The greatest enemy of a patient-centric perspective – once we acknowledge the collective nature of the patient and of self-care – is the tendency to freeze or fix the patient within a single definition, classification or perspective. When discussing the notion of infrastructure we underlined its excessive colonizing logic. In this concluding discussion, we wish to outline a general design principle that reflects our argument and might provide an alternative model for exploring these issues. We call this principle: the problem of fixing (in the sense of freezing) things. The researcher Annamarie Mol, mentioned earlier, provides a starting point for examining this problem (2008). According to her, fixing things would frustrate the possibility to explore, and to experiment, and provide space for attuning the various "viscous variables" relevant in caring for each other. In other words, fixing things frustrates the collective learning process around the experience of the disease. Mol notes:

> " The logic of choice suggests that choosing is confined to specific moments. Privileged moments, difficult maybe, but bounded. The logic of care, by contrast, suggests that attuning the many viscous variables of a life to each other is a continuing process. It goes on and on, until the day you die." (2008)

The notion of building an infrastructure, by contrast, requires us to fix things and thus does not allow for continuous learning as stated above. In this way, delicate, unstable and extremely complex situations will be condensed, alternatives will be measured, and a solution determined through evidence produced in a laboratory (evidence that often has little to do with the daily aspects of dealing with the disease). Mol argues that patients and their bodies should not be trapped in causal chains and pre-formatted paths. Rather, they are embedded in treatment practices: *Practices designed to foster 'patient choice' erode existing practices that were established to ensure 'good care'.* As she eloquently notes:

> "Care is a process: it does not have clear boundaries. It is open-ended. Care is not a transaction in which something is exchanged (a product against a price); but an interaction in which the action goes back and forth (in an ongoing process)....care is an iterative, open-ended process that might be shaped and reshaped depending on its results..." (Mol, 2008)

Infrastructuring patient self-care into the larger healthcare system runs the risk of making too cramped a space for the patient. It might alter daily practices in ways that do not necessarily fit well with the intricacies of the disease from a patient-centric view. Rather than becoming part of an infrastructure, patients might wish to have opportunities for empowering themselves through the use of platforms for care where care is still seen as an open-ended collective process, and expertise is democratized and negotiable. In this sense, we might wish to rebalance the dominant and central position of the biomedical discourse and therefore design spaces for doctors to learn a bit more about their patients and their experiences, while also allowing patients to better relate to doctors' concerns. The focus should be on maximizing social learning and not simply minimizing costs, as we have come to learn that interventions focused on saving costs often end up establishing more sophisticated interventions where costs actually increase (refer back to our first vignette). In this sense, the positivistic and value-free position of biomedical reductionism inscribed in the super-structure might just act as a barrier to new ways of thinking about the production and design of medical knowledge and technology. Obviously, we do not want to completely erase the medical model in health and self-care but to point to its intrinsic limits, its tendency to overlook aspects that, we believe, are relevant in a patient-centric perspective, and even more relevant when it comes to the design of self-care support systems.

A Plea for Modest Technology, *Hybrid Forums* and *Open-Ended Doctoring*

We would like to conclude our argument by briefly noting possible directions for future study – exploring concepts and design spaces which might open up our thinking about future self-care platforms, where the self is not studied in isolation, and not constrained by an imposed discourse. Among the many alternative frameworks being proposed, we find that approaches in science and technology studies research and policy studies seem to us the most apt and inspiring. We point to three concepts that represent new starting points for thinking of alternative models: Jasanoff's notion of a *technology of humility*, Callon's concept of *hybrid forums* and Mol's ideas on *doctoring and patientism*.

Common to these three notions is the need for social and collective learning and a rejection of colonizing perspectives. Jasanoff (2003) critiques positivistic and predictive approaches and the technology that sustains them. It is in discussing the actual relation among decision-makers, experts, and citizens in the management of technology, that Jasanoff claims:

> *"Today, there is a need for 'technologies of humility' to complement the predictive approaches: to make apparent the possibility of unforeseen consequences; to make explicit the normative that lurks within the*

technical; and to acknowledge from the start the need for plural viewpoints and collective learning [...] The time is ripe for seriously re-evaluating existing models and approaches"

For her, a technology of humility is opposed to that of *hubris* inspired by the positivistic myth of progress, control and predictability. A technology of humility is instead constituted by

"methods, or better yet institutionalized habits of thought, that try to come to grips with the ragged fringes of human understanding – the unknown, the uncertain, the ambiguous, and the uncontrollable. Acknowledging the limits of prediction and control, technologies of humility confront 'head-on' the normative implications of our lack of perfect foresight" [pg. 227]

The dangers of certain infrastructure approaches is that we may end up working with (to use Jasanoff's words) *" conceptual models that seek to separate science from values, and that emphasize prediction and control at the expense of reflection and social learning. "*

In a similar vein, Callon et al. (2009) have recently introduced the concept of *Hybrid forum* as a way to extend traditional representative democracy (based on delegation) in favor of dialogical democracy. Discussions that occur in hybrid forums reframe the traditional asymmetry between experts and laypersons, whose separation is at the very centre of Callon's critique. The first aspect of hybrid forums is that we should accept the fact that the knowledge of specialists is not the only knowledge possible, and consequently we should recognize the richness and relevance of knowledge developed by laypersons who possess their own *capacity of diagnosis, an interpretation of the facts, a range of solutions*. In their illuminating work, the authors state that the traditional separation between experts and laypersons are outmoded.

Similar to Jasanoff, Callon et al. (2009) are seeking a notion that would foster dialogue and give voice to the variety of perspectives and forms of knowledge in play. The work of Mol (2008), which is more explicitly focused on the medical domain, reaffirms these points of Jasanoff and Callon. In an attempt to describe what would be a democratization of expertise in medicine, she introduces the notion of *doctoring* as central in the logic of care:

"A team that shares the task of doctoring offers an interesting model for the democratization of expertise. [...] The logic of care suggests a different way of opening up the monopoly of professional groups over

expertise.[...] creative practitioners (physicians, nurses, dieticians, physiotherapists, patients and patient groups) need time, money and space to experiment with innovations for daily care practices"

For Mol caring is in fact a matter of doctoring that, in her view, must be understood as a form of tinkering with bodies, technology and knowledge, – and with people too.

Thus doctoring and participating with modest technology in hybrid forums become for us the most interesting framework from which to examine emerging problems in our health care systems, to reflect on the role of technology, and therefore on our role as designers and developers.

REFERENCES

Anderson, Robert M. and Funnell, Martha M., (2000) Compliance and Adherence are Dysfunctional Concepts in Diabetes Care, *The Diabetes Educator*, 26; 597

Hilary Arksey and Patricia Sloper (1999) Disputed diagnoses: the cases of RSI and childhood cancer, *Social Science & Medicine*, vol. 49, no. 4, pp. 483-497

Barbot, Janine (2006) How to build an "active" patient? The work of AIDS associations in France, Social Science & Medicine 62 (2006) 538–551

Barry, Christine A., Bradley, Colin P., Britten, Nicky., Stevenson, Fione A., Barber, N. (2000) Patients'unvoiced agendas in general practice consultations: qualitative study, *British Medical Journal*, 320:1246-1250

Beisecker, Analee E. (1988). Aging and the desire for information and input in medical decisions: Patient consumerism in medical encounters, *The Gerontologist*, 28, 330–335

Berg, Marc (1999): Accumulating and Co-ordinating: Occasions for Information Technologies in Medical Work, *Journal of Computer Supported Cooperative Work,* vol. 8, pp. 373–401.

Berg, Marc and Timmermans, Stefan (2000), Orders and their Other: on the constitution of universalities in Medical Work, *Configuration*, vol. 8, 1, pp. 31-61

Borell, Merriley (1993) Training the senses, training the mind, in W.F. Bynum & R. Porter (eds), *Medicine and the five senses*. Cambridge, UK: Cambridge University Press, pp. 244-261.

Bowker, Geoffrey C. and Star, Susan L. (2000): *Sorting Things Out: Classification and its Consequences*, Cambridge, MIT press.

Britten, Nicky (1994) Patients' ideas about medicine: a qualitative study in a general practice population, *British Journal of General Practice*, 44, 465-468

Brown, Phil, McCormick, Sabrina, Mayer, Brian; Zavestoski, Stephen; Rachel Morello-Frosch, Rebecca Gasior Altman and Laura Senier, (2006) A Lab of Our Own": Environmental Causation of Breast Cancer and Challenges to the Dominant Epidemiological Paradigm, *Science Technology Human Values,* 31; 499

Brown, John S., Duguid, Paul (2000) *The Social Life of Information*, Boston: Harvard Business School Press

Cahill, Jack (1996) Patient participation: a concept analysis, *Journal of advanced nursing*, 24, pp. 561-71

Cahill, Jack (1998) Patient participation: a review of the literature, in *Journal of Clinical Nursing*, 7, 119-128

Callon, Micheal (1999) The Role of Lay People in the Production and Dissemination of Scientific Knowledge, *Science Technology & Society*, 4; 81

Callon, Michael, Lascoumes, Paul, Barthe, Yanic. (2009) *Acting in an Uncertain World: An Essay on Technical Democracy*, Cambridge, MIT press

Callon, Michael, and Rabeharisoa, Vololona (2003) research in the wild and the shaping of new social identities, in *Technology in Society*, Vol. 25, pp. 193-204

Ciborra Claudio, e Hanset, Hole (1999) From Tool to Gestell: Agendas for Managing the Information Infrastructure, *Information, Technology and People*, 11 (4): 305-327

Conrad, Peter (1985) The Meaning of Medications: Another Look at Compliance. *Social Science and Medicine*, vol. 20, pp. 29-37

Donovan Jenny L. and Blake, David R. (1992) Patient non-compliance: deviance or reasoned decision-making? *Social Science Medicine*, 34: 507-513.

Deveugele, Myriam, Anselm Derese, Atie van den Brink-Muinen, Jozien Bensing, Jan De Maeseneer (2002) Consultation length in general practice: cross sectional study in six European countries, *British Medicine Journal* 325:472

Edwards, Paul N., Bowker, Geoffrey C., Jackson, Steven J., Williams, Robin (2009) Introduction: An Agenda for Infrastructure Studies, *Journal of the Association of Information Systems*, 10, Special Issue, pp. 364-374

Ellingsen, Gunnar and Monteiro, Eric (2006) Seamless Integration: Standardization across Multiple local settings, *Journal of Computer Supported Cooperative Work*, vol. 15, pp. 443-466

Foucault, Michael (1973) *The Birth of the Clinic*, London, Tavistock

Fitzpatrick, Geraldine (2004) Integrated care and the working record, *Health Informatics Journal*, vol. 10, pp. 291- 304

Goguen, Joseph (2005) Support for Ontological Diversity and Evolution, short essay for the *SEEK (Science Environment for Ecological Knowledge)* project meeting, October 27. Available at:
http://www.cs.ucsd.edu/users/goguen/papers/onto-intgn.html

Hanseth, Ole, Thoresen, Kari and Winner, Langdon (1993) The Politics of Networking Technology in Health Care, *Journal of Computer Supported Cooperative Work*, vol. 2, no. 2.

Hanseth, Ole and Braa, Christine (2001) Hunting for the treasure at the end of the rainbow: standardizing corporate IT infrastructures, *Journal of Computer Supported Cooperative Work*, vol 10, no. 3-4, pp. 261-292

Hanseth, Ole and Lundberg, Nina (2001) Design work oriented infrastructure, *Journal of Computer Supported Cooperative Work*, vol. 10, no. 3-4, pp. 347-372

Hardey, Michael (2001) E'Health: the internet and the transformation of patients into consumer and producers of Health Knowledge, *Information, communication and society*, 4(3): 388-40

Hartsock, Nancy, CM. (1998) *The feminist standpoint revisited and other essays*, Perseus Publishing

Heath, Christian (1992) The delivery and reception of diagnosis in the general-practice consultation. In Drew, P. and Heritage, J. (eds) *Talk at Work: Interaction in Institutional Settings,* Cambridge: Cambridge University Press

Helman Cecil G. (1981) 'Tonic', 'fuel' and 'food': social and symbolic aspects of the long-term use of psychotropic drugs, *Social Science Medicine*, 15B: 521-533.

Hewison, Alistair 1995 Nurses' power in interactions with patients *Journal of Advanced Nursing*, vol. 21 no. 1, pp. 75 - 82

Jasanoff, Sheila (2003) Technology of Humility, in *Minerva*, 41, 223-244

Jirotka, Marina, Procter, Rob, Hartswood, Marc, Slack, Roger, Simpson, Andrew and Voss Alex (2005) Collaboration and Trust in Healthcare

Innovation: The eDiaMoND Case study, *Journal of Computer Supported Cooperative Work*, vol. 14, pp. 369-398

Jones David R. (1979) Drugs and prescribing: what the patient thinks, *Journal of general practice*, 29, 417-419.

Kamel Boulos, Maged, N., and Wheelert, Steve (2007) The emerging Web 2.0 social software: an enabling suite of sociable technologies in health and health care education, *Health Information and Libraries Journal*, 24, 2-23

Knorr-Cetina, Karin, (1999) *Epistemic Cultures: How the Sciences Make Knowledge.* Harvard University Press, Cambridge

Kilbourn, Kyle (2008) *The Patient as skilled practitioner. A design anthropology approach to enskilment in Health and Technology.* PhD dissertation, Mads Clausen Institute for Product Innovation, University of Southern Denmark

Lachmund, Jens (1997) *Der abgehorte Koerper, Zur historischen Soziologie der medizinischen Untersuchung*, Westdeutscher, Verlag

Leder, Drew (1992) A tale of two bodies: The Cartesian corpse and the lived body, Leder, D. (ed), *The Body in Medical Thought and Practice*, Amsterdam: Kluwer Academic Publishers

Levenstein Joseph H., McCracken, Eric C., McWhinney, Ian, Steward, Moira A. and Brown, Judith B. (1986) The patient-centred clinical method: a model for the doctor-patient interaction in family medicine, *Family Practice*, 3:24-30

Nettleton, S and Burrows, R., (2003) E-Scaped Medicine? Information, Reflexivity and Health. Critical Social Policy, 23(2), 165-185

Martin, David, Hartwood, Mark, Slack Roger and Voss, Alex (2006) Achieving Dependability in the Configuration, Integration and testing of Healthcare Technologies, *Journal of Computer Supported Cooperative Work*, vol. 15, pp. 467-499

Macintyre, Sally and Oldman, David (1977) Coping with migraine. In Davis, A. and Horobin, G. (eds) *Medical encounters: the experience of illness and treatment*, London: Croom Helm

Morgan Myfanwy and Watkins C.J. (1988) Managing hypertension: beliefs and responses to medication among cultural groups. *Social Health Illness*, 10: 561-578.

Mol, Annamarie (2008) *The logic of care and the problem of patient choice*, London Routledge

Molzahn, Anita E. (1991) Quality of life after organ transplantation, *Journal of advanced nursing*, vol. 16, no. 9, pp. 1042-7

Morgan, Myfanwy and Watkins, Carol J. (1988) Managing hypertension: beliefs and responses to medication among cultural groups, *Sociology of Health & Illness* vol. 10, no. 4, pp. 561-578

Opie, Anne (1998) 'Nobody asked me for my view': Users' empowerment by multidisciplinary health teams, *Qualitative health research*, vol. 8, no. 2, pp.188-206

Osterberg, Lars and Blaschke, Terrence (2005) Adherence to medication, *New England Journal of Medicine*, 353(5), 487-97

Pinelle, David and Gutwin, Carl (2006) Loose coupling and Health Care organizations, *Journal of Computer Supported Cooperative Work*, vol. 15, no. 5-6, pp. 537-572

Pipek, Volkmar and Wulf, Volker (2009) Infrastructuring: toward an integrated perspective on the design and use of Information Technology, *Journal of the association of Information systems,* vol. 10, Special Issue, pp. 447-473

Procter, Rob, Rouncefield, Mark, Balka, Hellen and Berg, Marc (2006) Special Issue: CSCW ad Dependable Healthcare Systems, *Journal of Computer Supported Cooperative Work*, vol. 15, pp. 413-418

Paterson, Barbara (2001) The myth of patient empowerment in chronic illness, *Journal of advance nursing* 34(5), 574-581

Pilnick, Alison (1998) 'Why didn't you say just that?' Dealing with issue of asymmetry, knowledge and competence in the pharmacist/client encounter, *Sociology of Health and Illness*, 20(1), 29-51

Preece, Jenny (1998) Empatic communities: reaching out across the web, in *Interaction*, march+april

Rabeharisoa, Vololona and Callon, Michael (1998) The participation of patients in the process of production of knowledge: the case of the french muscular distrophies association, *Sciences Sociales et Santé*, vol. 16, 3, pp. 41

Rabeharisoa, Vololona and Callon, Micheal (2002) The involvement of patients' associations in research, *International Social Science Journal*, Vol. 54, 171, pp. 57 – 63

Rabeharisoa. Vololona, Callon. Michael (2004) Patients and scientists French muscular dystrophy research, in Jasanoff, S. (ed.), *States of knowledge*, London, Routledge

Radley, Alan (1994) *Making Sense of Illness: The Social Psychology of Health and Disease*. London: Sage

Reddy, Madhu C., Dourish, Paul and Pratt, Wanda (2006) Temporality in Medical Work: Time also Matters, *Journal Computer Supported Cooperative Work*, vol. 15, pp. 29-53

Ribes, David and Finholt, Thimas, A. (2009) The long now of technology infrastructure: articulating tensions in development, *Journal of the association of Information systems*, 10, Special Issue, pp. 376-398

Roberson, Mildred H. B. (1992), The Meaning of Compliance: Patient Perspectives, *Qualitative Health Research*, Vol. 2, No. 1, 7-26

Schneider, Karin and Wagner, Ina (1993): Constructing the 'Dossier Repre´sentatif': Computer-Based Information Sharing in French Hospitals, *Journal of Computer Supported Cooperative Work*, vol. 2, no. 1, pp. 229–253

Schmidt, Kield and Simone, Carla (1996): Coordination Mechanisms: Towards a Conceptual Foundation of CSCW Systems Design, *Journal of Computer Supported Cooperative Work*, 5:155–

Star, Susan L. (1999) 'The Ethnography of Infrastructure', *American Behavioral Scientist* 43: 377-91.

Star, Susan L. and Ruhleder, Karen (1996) Steps Towards an Ecology of Infrastructure: Design and Access for Large Information Spaces, *Information Systems Research*, vol. 7, no. 1, pp. 111–134.

Star, Susan L. and Bowker, Geoffrey (2002) "How to infrastructure," in Lievrouw L. A. and Livingstone, S. (Eds.) *Handbook of New Media - Social Shaping and Consequences of ICTs*, London, SAGE, pp. 151-162.

Suchman, Lucy (1994) Do categories have politics? *Journal of Computer supported cooperative work*, vol. 2, no. 3, pp. 177-190

Turner, Bryan S. (1987) *Medical Power and Social Knowledge*, London, Sage

Turner, William, Bowker, Geoffrey, Gasser, Les and Zackland Manuel (2006) Information Infrastructure for distributed collective practices, *Journal of Computer Supported Cooperative Work*, Vol. 15, Special issue 2-3, pp. 93-110

Ure, Jenny, Hartswood, Mark, Wardlaw, Joanna, Procter, Rob, Anderson, Stuart, Gonzalez-Velez, Horacio, Lin, Yu-wei, Lloyd, Sharon, Ho, Kate (2009) The development of data infrastructure of e-Health: a socio-technical perspective, *Journal of the association of Information systems*, 10, Special Issue, pp. 415-429

Verbeek-Heida Piet M. (1992) How patients look at drug therapy: consequences for therapy negotiations in medical consultations. *Family Practice*, 10: 326-329.

Winthereik, Brit R. and Vikkelso, Signe (2005) ICT and Integrated Care: Some dilemmas of standardising Inter-Organisational Communication, *Journal of Computer Supported Cooperative Work*, vol. 14, pp. 42-67

INDEX

I

J

T

U